BY MICHAEL OLAJIDE, JR.

Aerobox®

SLEEKIFY!™

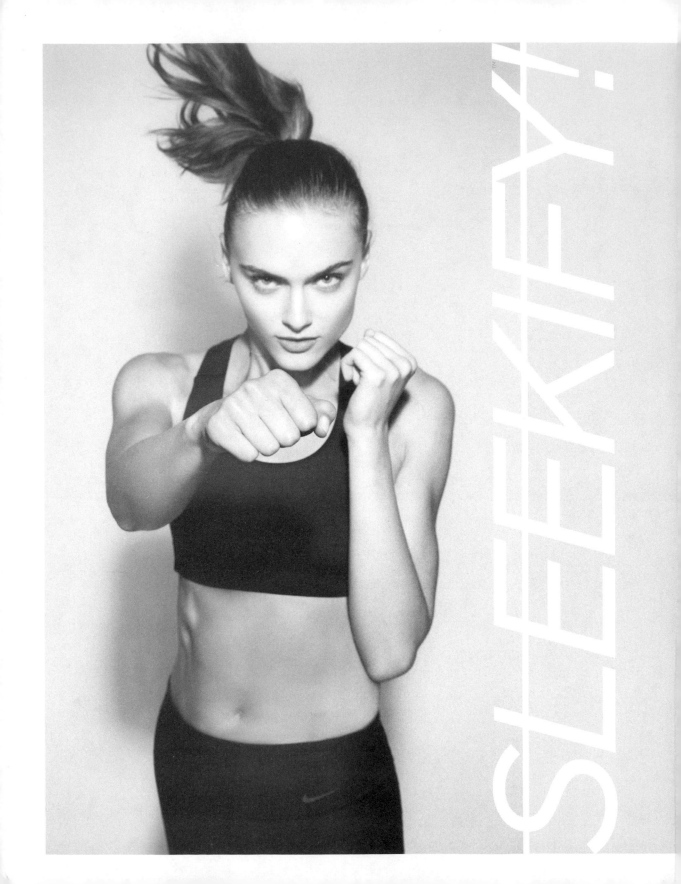

SLEEKIFY!™

THE SUPERCHARGED NO-WEIGHTS WORKOUT TO SCULPT AND TIGHTEN YOUR BODY IN 28 DAYS!

MICHAEL OLAJIDE, JR.,

WITH MYATT MURPHY

FOREWORD BY **ADRIANA LIMA**

Z

ZINC INK

BALLANTINE BOOKS

NEW YORK

This book proposes a program of diet and exercise recommendations for the reader to follow. However, you should consult a qualified medical professional (and, if you are pregnant, your ob/gyn) before starting this or any other fitness program. Please seek your doctor's advice before making any decisions that affect your health or extreme changes in your diet, particularly if you suffer from any medical condition or have any symptom that may require treatment. As with any diet or exercise program, if at any time you experience any discomfort, stop immediately and consult your physician.

A Zinc Ink Trade Paperback Original

Copyright © 2013 by Michael Olajide, Jr.

Published in the United States by Zinc Ink,
an imprint of The Random House Publishing Group,
a division of Random House LLC,
a Penguin Random House Company, New York.

BALLANTINE and the HOUSE colophon are
registered trademarks of Random House, Inc.

ZINC INK is a trademark of Galvanized Brands, LLC.

SLEEKIFY! is a trademark of Michael Olajide, Jr.

AEROBOX is a registered trademark of Total Eclipse Enterprises Inc.

AEROSCULPT and AEROJUMP are trademarks of Michael Olajide, Jr.

AEROSPACE HIGH PERFORMANCE CENTER is a registered
trademark of Aerofox LLC DBA Aerospace High Performance Center.

ISBN 978-0-345-54967-9

eBook ISBN 978-0-345-54968-6

Printed in the United States of America

www.ballantinebooks.com

2 4 6 8 9 7 5 3 1

Photographs by Ben Watts
Book design by Barbara M. Bachman

In this book I dedicate my efforts to Dr. A. Alessandro Pireno,
the father of my rebirth and forever in my daily thoughts

FOREWORD

BABY WEIGHT TO RUNWAY WEIGHT—
IN FIVE WEEKS!

N SEPTEMBER 2012, MY HUSBAND, MARKO, AND I WERE LUCKY ENOUGH TO HAVE OUR second daughter, Sienna.

Yet just eight weeks after I gave birth to Sienna, I had to step onto the stage of the Victoria's Secret Fashion Show, under the bright lights of the runway, in nothing but a bra, panties . . . and angel's wings. The show is my absolute favorite event of the year, and Victoria's Secret has given me so many opportunities in my life that I knew I had to be sexy, sleek, and baby-weight-free—there was no other option. Suddenly, the pressure was on and I was so nervous and scared! I had to get my body back, and there was only one person to call: my trainer, my good friend, Michael Olajide, Jr.

Three weeks after Sienna was born, my doctor gave me the okay to start working out again. That meant I had only five weeks to get back into Victoria's Secret Angel shape and be ready to represent the sexiest, most beautiful lingerie brand in the world.

I started working out with Michael every single day, until the day before the show. His boxing-inspired workouts were exactly what I needed to get on the runway with a beautiful, flat stomach, great legs, and tons of confidence.

The Sleekify fitness program gets you looking great from every angle: Shadow boxing, jumping rope and rope combinations, and low-weight-bearing exercises are the perfect combination for a sleek, fit body. Training like a boxer gave me a "fighter's mind," as Michael calls it, and the confidence to realize that losing forty pounds of baby weight in the very short period of time before the show was completely possible, with the right training and dedication.

What I love most about his method of training is that it is different every time we do it, which keeps it exciting. It is convenient, too: The jumping rope, which is *my* favorite secret tool, I love because I can fit in a workout at home while my little girls are napping.

I also love that my upper body, core, and lower body are pushed to their limits with little to no weight—and all the boxing combinations keep my heart rate up, so the effects of the workout continue long after we have set down the jump rope and taken off the gloves. That means I always have to step it up. Every session is a challenge—and anyone who knows me well can tell you that I love a great challenge!

After a couple of weeks of really hard work, the pregnancy weight I had gained started to come right off. My body was working hard to keep up with the high-intensity workouts; I began shedding the pounds, more every day.

Of course, I was on an incredibly clean diet, too, based on Sleekify guidelines, with lots of protein, few carbs, and plenty of water. Michael motivated me through every step of this challenge. He treated me like a boxing champion preparing for a fight. He never let me give up or slack off. We pushed every single day. I love that intensity!

By the night before the show, I had met the challenge. Stepping onto that stage again with all the other beautiful Victoria's Secret Angels, lights shining and millions of viewers watching my every move, I felt incredible. Everyone could see that I was back. My body felt so sleek and balanced, and my energy was through the roof!

I could not have done any of it without Michael, who has given me his very best tools to get incredibly fit and stay gorgeous anytime, anywhere, through Sleekify.

You do not have to be a supermodel, or a boxer, or a professional athlete, to experience the effects of this amazing program. You just have to want to look great, feel great, and perform at your very best.

—Adriana Lima

CONTENTS

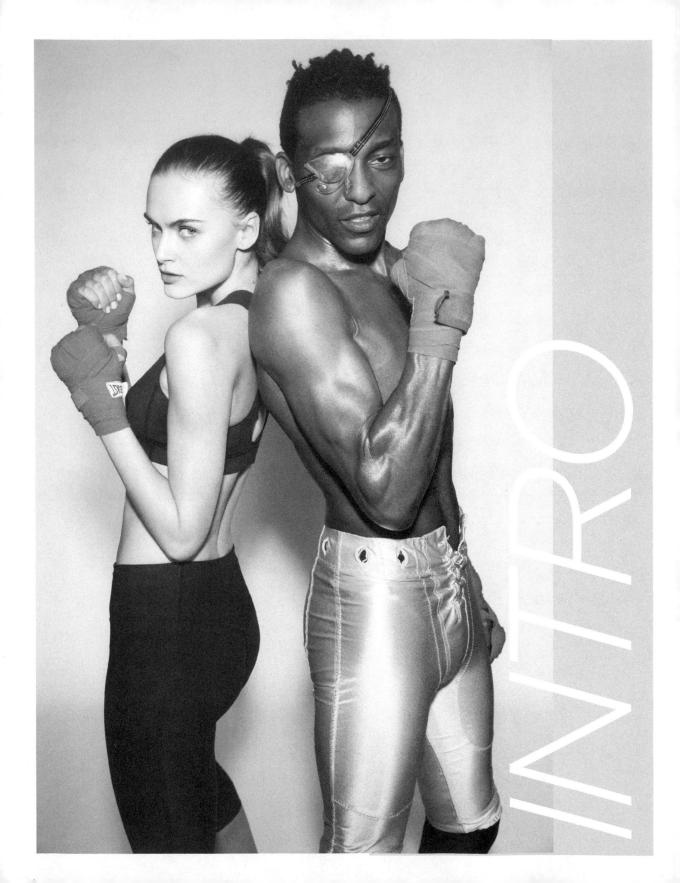

INTRO

INTRODUCTION

O NLY ONE PERSON CAN COME BETWEEN YOU AND THE BODY YOU'VE ALWAYS wanted. And that person is you.

You are your only opponent, and getting into the best shape of your life is a constant fight—a fight between who you are today and who you want to be tomorrow. But now you're not alone in that fight. With this book in hand, you have a secret plan, an effective and proven program, and someone unique in your corner: me.

When a boxer returns to his (or her!) corner, it's his entourage that not only reminds him of the techniques he needs to employ to win, but pumps him up so that he realizes how great he is and how strong he is. It's these "cornermen" who make a boxer feel as if he can't be defeated.

Well, I'm your cornerman now. And I'm here to get you in shape for the next big moment of your life.

It might be an upcoming wedding, a high school reunion, or having to bare all on the beach while on vacation. Or—if you're like my clients—it could be to turn every head on the runway or at a big movie premiere. Or maybe you've simply had enough with what you see in the mirror and you're finally ready to earn what you deserve.

No matter what your reason may be, when the clock is ticking and you need to be in the best shape possible—in as little time as possible—it takes a carefully designed routine to melt away those pounds and transform your body into one worth showing off.

Well, congratulations, because that's what you're holding in your hands. Getting people into the best shape of their lives is what I do for a living. I'm the best at it, because my life and the livelihoods of my clients depend on it.

That's Sleekify—a culmination of everything I've used with my clients over the past twenty years to help them achieve the sleek, powerfully fit, and well-defined body of a top-level athlete.

Sleekify is more than a calorie-blasting, heart-pumping program that burns more than a thousand calories a session, attacks fat, and sculpts seriously lean muscle in record time. It's a unique and truly authentic physical and mental training program. Every single move—every punch, jump, exercise, and drill you'll do throughout the entire twenty-eight-day plan—has a specific purpose.

It's not faux boxing. It's not throwing punches for the purpose of throwing punches. There's nothing that disturbs me, a former championship boxer myself, more than seeing someone teach a fake rendition of something steeped in such history and mystique. I could never do such a disservice to such a noble sport. Instead, each punch, each head movement, and every combination means something—and will *do* something for your body—because every single thing about Sleekify is real. It follows the same exact disciplines that boxers use to prepare their bodies for every possible contingency. But more important, it's the program I use with all of my clients.

Many of my clients aren't allowed to have "pretty good" bodies, because that's not what they're hired for. Instead, they have to have exceptional bodies that are "show-ready" at all times because their career may depend on it. Your paycheck may not depend on looking your absolute best, but that doesn't mean you aren't capable of feeling that same pressure when standing in front of the mirror.

What Sleekify does—and why it works for men and women alike—is that it amplifies what's underneath. A body reflects what it does, and if you put it in the atmosphere of doing something quick, light, highly repetitive, but challenging to your muscles from head to toe—it will reflect that. The Sleekify program cuts away the excess, leaving behind the reflection of a healthier, leaner, sculpted body of celebrity proportions.

Like I said before, it's the choices we make and the effort we put into them that decide how our story ends. And this is your opportunity to have your story end exactly the way you've always wanted it to—with you as a winner.

When I teach, my goal is to make sure every single individual who comes into my class leaves fitter than when they came in. I do that because I believe there is a winner inside all of us, and I know that everyone has her or his own personal fight. It's a fight they can win, but only if they are shown the right way to do it.

You are your only opponent. And right now, it's time to start fighting for the body you deserve. And know that from this moment on, you're never alone. I'll be your trainer now. I'll be your cornerman, because there's only one thing I love more than teaching the gift of fitness: watching people succeed with fitness.

With Sleekify, you will succeed—by doing nothing more than simply trying your best.

SLEEKIFY!™

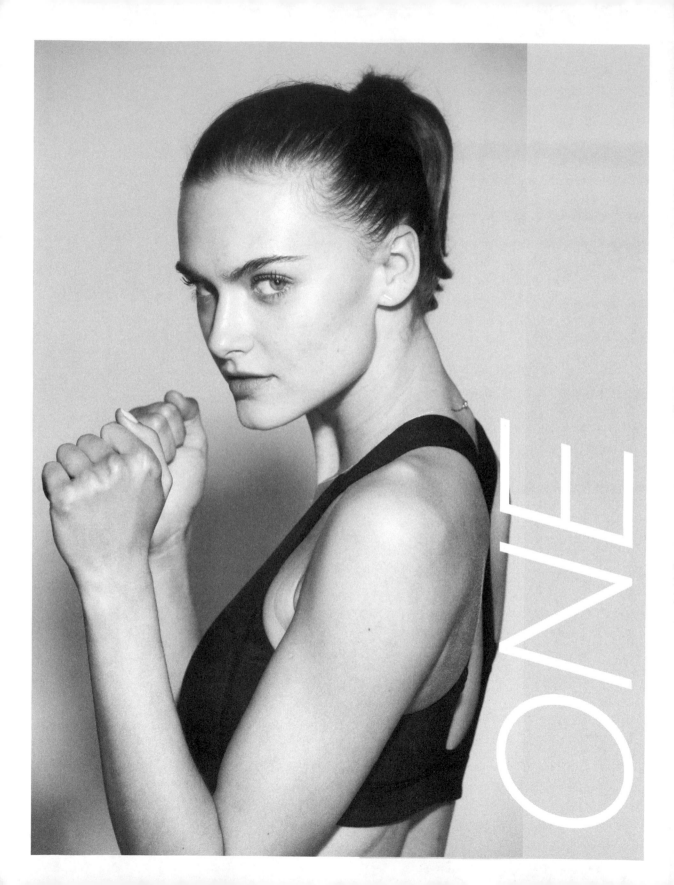

THE SECRET
OF SLEEK

BEFORE I CO-FOUNDED AEROSPACE HIGH PERFORMANCE CENTER IN NEW YORK City and became known for my intense workout classes . . . Before I started training everyone from average housewives and senior citizens to supermodels and celebrities, including Hugh Jackman, Eva Mendes, and 50 Cent . . . Before I taught classes that were attended by everyone from Mary J. Blige to James Taylor . . . Before the world took notice when I helped Victoria's Secret Angel Adriana Lima lose all of her post-pregnancy weight so she was slim, sleek, and show-ready in just five weeks . . .

Before every opportunity I've ever been blessed with throughout my twenty-plus-year career in fitness, I was a boxer. In fact, by the time I was twenty-two, I was just one fight away from accomplishing my life's dream of becoming the International Boxing Federation Middleweight Champion of the World. But if you think I'm sharing my boxing past because I want to impress you with my successes, you would be absolutely wrong.

Instead, I hope to inspire you through my losses.

MY STORY

My signature eye patch isn't a fashion statement. Instead, it covers up an injury that closed the door on my professional fighting career forever, and opened the door to the fitness career I've enjoyed for two decades. It also reminds me every day about something I believe in quite strongly.

Sometimes, the stories that end positively are the ones that are born from something negative. It's through the choices we make—and the effort we put into those choices—that we decide how our own story ends.

I was fifteen, living in Vancouver, British Columbia, with my mom, when my sister reminded me that my dad—a former pro boxer—had a gym where he trained fighters, and suggested I try the sport. At the time, I really didn't know what I wanted to do with my life, but I had always been mesmerized by the spirit, athleticism, and abilities of boxers like Muhammad Ali, Joe Frazier, and George Foreman.

When I went to live and train with my dad, my career left the ground pretty fast. By the time I turned eighteen in 1981, with less than a year and a half of amateur boxing under my belt, I was ready to go pro. Four years later, I earned a contract with Madison Square Garden, found myself ranked among the top fifteen middleweight contenders worldwide, and moved to New York City to fulfill my dream.

I was undefeated and only a few fights away from a title bout when I took an uppercut to my right eye while sparring. The punch hit me so hard, it destroyed the orbital floor in my face, causing what some call a bombardier fracture—or a permanent drop of the eye within its socket.

I continued to fight—and win—and eventually became the number-one middleweight contender in the world, despite the fact that I was suffering from double vision and depth perception issues. But the reality at that point was that my journey to become world champion had become a whole lot harder.

I wouldn't realize until fighting junior middleweight Olympic gold medalist Frank Tate for the middleweight title in 1987 that my dream would be impossible.

We fought that night for fifteen rounds, and I remember feeling drained and lethargic, even though I'd been training hard for the bout. I remember being very aware of everything around me, which is unusual for a fighter when they're focused and the adrenaline is flowing. But that night, I could hear the crowd. I could even hear people talking. And I could feel every single punch. Being in that place—having that lack of focus—is never a good place for anyone to be, whether you're a fighter, another sort of athlete, or anyone with a goal that needs to be achieved.

I went into the ring that night undefeated, but came out suffering my first loss by decision—one that wouldn't be my last. As my vision grew worse, I became legally blind in my right eye; I eventually had to retire in 1991 with a record of 28-4, twenty by knockout. I was twenty-six years old, still physically in my prime, and my career ended as quickly as it began—like a flash.

But losing my vision only gave me focus in another direction.

Although I could no longer compete, I knew I could still maintain the same physique, the same low body-fat level, the same sleekness of muscle, and the same fast reflexes using a boxing-based program of exercises and maneuvers. The same exercises and maneuvers that I—as well as every single fighter who has ever come before me or comes after me—rely on to get my body in the best shape possible.

FOR ME, WEIGHT LOSS has never been an issue, but for most everyone that I've worked with over the years, it's a major problem.

I sometimes will hear others say that the reason certain people—such as athletes, models, and naturally slim individuals—may never struggle with weight loss issues is because they're born with a fast metabolism: a supercharged metabolism that burns fat faster all day long and lets them eat more calories—and any type of food they want—without ever having to worry about packing on the pounds.

Is it true that some people are born with faster-than-normal metabolisms that burn calories more quickly so they store less body fat? Absolutely. But if you think that every athlete and every professional model has an amazing physique because they're all blessed with a one-of-a-kind metabolism, that's where you would be wrong.

I can honestly say that a lot of my clients—men and women with sculpted, lean, Sleekified bodies who appear to have naturally turbo-charged fat-burning furnaces—actually have normal metabolisms. In fact, some—and I mean celebrities with the most enviable bodies imaginable—have very slow metabolisms that are most likely less revved than your own.

Don't believe me? Do you still think they are superhuman? Then just take a look at a lot of athletes after they retire or watch what happens when your favorite actor or actress is in between jobs. Many lose their physiques. They may have incredible bodies when they're active in their sport or preparing for a role or a big runway show, but when the spotlight is off, you can see just how human we all can be.

Stars aren't all genetically superior to the rest of us—their physiques are a result of the work they're willing to put into themselves and the investment they make in themselves. They could continue to have those physiques if they continued to work at it, but once they stop getting paid to be in their best shape possible, many lack the motivation to bother. In other words, they give up the fight.

As for me, I don't work out at the same intense level that I used to when I was fighting professionally in my early twenties, and I may no longer have the same physical abilities, either. But I do have a sleeker body now than when I was that age.

The aging process may be inevitable, and everyone has his or her own unique physical makeup and metabolism. But no matter what type of physique you're currently saddled with or how old you may be, you can recalibrate your metabolism—and teach your body to burn calories faster and more efficiently—by altering how you exercise and the amount of calories you consume. It really is *that* simple.

WHY OTHER PROGRAMS FAIL

Every week, there seems to be something new in terms of diet and exercise. Some new way to lose weight and get healthy that's better than the one before it. There are a million different options out there. And there's a reason for all those confusing choices.

It's our nature as human beings to look for the quick fix and to seek out that which is most convenient. But the problem with most fad diets and flash-in-the-pan workout routines is that they have no substance or foundation.

Most so-called brand-new exercise routines, classes, DVDs, or fitness products might say they are able to "blast more fat" or "build more muscle," but these same products also promise that you can do all of this without having to put in as much time or effort compared to other workouts. Just that promise alone—the offer to help you accomplish everything by putting in zero to little effort—should be an immediate red flag that warns you that what you will achieve is far from what they claim to offer.

Many fad diets are no better, usually based around whatever new fat-loss study or health trend is popular at that moment, such as sticking with a gluten-free diet, eating for your blood type, or matching the foods you eat with your pH levels, for example. But look behind the curtain and chances are, the program many of these diets recommend is the same basic workout plan and low-calorie diet. It's not new, and it's not better—it's just a different way of presenting the same type of program that didn't work last time you tried it, under a different name.

But there is no quick fix. Most of those so-called new options are nothing distractions that are keeping you from Sleekifying yourself. For something to work, it has to be realistic, it has to have a strong foundation, and it has to be something that can be sustained. It needs to be something that can fit into and complement your lifestyle, something powerful enough to change the unhealthy habits that you may already have, and something you can do for the rest of your life.

That's the power of Sleekify, a high-intensity, full-body, excuse-proof program that requires very little space or equipment—so you always have the means to work out—while it honestly targets more muscle fibers than the average exercise routine (so you always burn more fat and build more lean muscle). But best of all, it incorporates proven techniques that aren't today's new fad—they are the same time-tested exercises that have never failed to get boxers in the best shape of their lives. With Sleekify, you finally have the formula—and the foundation—your body has been waiting for.

The Exercise Enigma

For me, cardiovascular (or aerobic) exercise—any activity that increases your heart rate and elevates your body's consumption of oxygen—is king. Compared to strength training, flexibility, balance, and coordination exercise, cardio is the most important of all the fitness elements, which is why it accounts for about three-quarters of the Sleekify workout.

Not only is it the most effective tool for burning off fat, but performing the right amount of cardio each week can also help you live a healthier, longer life by improving your cholesterol numbers, strengthening your heart, and even lowering your blood pressure, among other equally important benefits.

So why isn't everyone using it to become sleeker? Most people tend to take two approaches when it comes to cardio and weight loss. One: They choose an activity that doesn't have a high enough intensity to achieve the results they hope to gain (for example, walking). Two: They think the answer lies in sticking with one activity—such as pedaling on a bike or running on a treadmill—until all of their unwanted weight drops off.

This can fail because most of the aerobic activities average people choose—running, cycling, or stair climbing, for example—target only certain, but not all, the muscles of the lower body (primarily legs, gluteal muscles, and calves). By using only your legs, you end up missing out on toning and training half of your body. That one-sided solution can leave you too tired with fewer results to show for all your hard work—or worse, cause chronic pain or an injury that could keep you from exercising altogether.

Building more lean muscle through resistance training also plays a key role in weight loss, since the more lean muscle you have, the higher you'll raise your resting metabolic rate (the amount of calories that your body burns all day long, even when at rest). The problem is that many of these catch-all programs are designed in a way that mostly exhausts the vanity muscles—the muscles you can see in the mirror, such as your chest, shoulders, and the front of your thighs (quadriceps)—while ignoring other equally important muscle groups because they're smaller, less sexy, or unseen (such as your calves, lower back, and hamstrings).

Resistance training programs also come with a number of expectations. They expect you to be able to invest in weights, equipment, mats, benches, and other tools you may not have room or money for, or to join and travel to a gym many times a week. They expect you to be at a certain fitness level, which may be too advanced or too basic to be effective for you right now. They never account for who you are and what you might or might not have, which is why many people find themselves on the receiving end of being excessively sore—or worse, constantly injured—as a result of lifting weights improperly. They also expect that you'll have access to a spotter—a person who can step in and assist you when your muscles tire out and can no longer lift the weight.

WHY SLEEKIFY SUCCEEDS

Sleekify is a methodology that's not too terribly different from yoga or tai chi. In fact, sometimes I refer to my program as "American Yoga" or the "Western Hemisphere's martial art."

Just as yoga and tai chi are disciplines that allow you to have a full range of motion, core control, and functional strength throughout most of your natural life, Sleekify offers the same lifetime guarantee because it's rooted in the sport of boxing and adapted to benefit the human body.

The exercises and maneuvers used in Sleekify are the same tried-and-true techniques that have been used by boxers since the sport's conception. That's why Sleekify remains just as effective and relevant today as it was when I first conceived many of the principles of the program two decades ago.

But what separates Sleekify from other fitness boxing workouts—and this is coming from a guy who was hailed as the "godfather of boxing fitness" two decades ago—is how you have complete control over its intensity. Sleekify is a combination of proven drills, advanced techniques, and unique body-sculpting exercises that adapts to your skill set, giving you back as much as you're willing to put into it—so you dictate the pace of your results.

What I've done with Sleekify is translate proven boxing methods into something people can understand and apply in their everyday lives. Sleekify works *for* every body because it's designed to work *with* your body, taking the same rooted principles of boxing and molding them into a routine that an ordinary individual, a high-performance athlete, or even a supermodel can use.

It doesn't convolute or take away from your body—but enhances it.

It allows anyone not pleased with their own physique to get back to their most primal and natural state by stripping away the fat and uncovering every individual muscle underneath. By the time you're finished with Sleekify, there's no excess—it's all been whittled away. It allows you to realize your full potential and see the sculpture that each of us has hidden beneath the surface.

And best of all, you don't need a class, a trainer, or a punching bag hanging from your basement ceiling. All you need is a little time and the will to win.

Whether you have a few pounds to lose, or ten, twenty, thirty, forty pounds, or beyond—the effects will almost seem instantaneous. But that's not the only way Sleekify will turn you into a winner.

Sleekify Leaves No One Behind

Have you ever tried running with a friend who was either less fit than you, or worse, was in better shape?

If so, then odds are you've either had to slow down to a pace that's less effective for you or speed up to a pace your body may not be ready to handle in order to exercise together. Resistance training with a friend can cause a similar issue, since it forces you to waste time having to constantly change how much weight you're lifting to accommodate for someone who may not be as strong as you (or is stronger than you).

Sleekify is unique in that the benefit you get is all in the effort you put into it. It focuses on what's inside you and your own abilities, so that both men and women—ranging from average beginners to elite athletes—can use the program right alongside one another. It's an even playing field that allows everybody to get 100 percent from it.

That's why when I teach my classes, my studio is always filled with an eclectic mix of people. Look in any direction and you'll find supermodels sweating it out next to seventy-year-old business executives. You'll see former athletes putting themselves through the paces as well as the average Joe who may be starting a workout regime for the very first time in his life. The reason they're able to exercise together is that my workout is designed so you always train at your own level—a level where you can expect to advance fairly quickly.

You may make quicker and bigger strides using the program than the person next to you, but with Sleekify, the fight is, and will always be, with yourself. That's why no matter how out of shape or fit you are, if you move as prescribed, you will win, and you'll see results almost immediately.

Sleekify Treats All Your Muscles Equally

I have never taken a single day off from teaching my classes since becoming a fitness professional in 1991. Part of that is because I never tire of teaching—I love the process! But it's also because thanks to this program, my body is so evenly balanced, I'm able to teach every day—sometimes up to six sessions daily—without ever worrying about it breaking down on me.

When most people think boxing, they associate the sport with getting injured. That's a reality when you're in the ring, or training improperly using some knockoff "boxing fitness" routine that doesn't focus on using proper form. But because Sleekify is a non-weight-bearing routine that hits all of your muscles from front to back and top to bottom, it's a more even workout that prevents you from pulling a muscle or overtraining a certain body part. It's a muscular balance that will prevent you from needing to take any downtime recovering from unnecessary injuries.

Sleekify and Never Crunch Again

Do you want to see your abs? If you can't right now, it's not because you're not doing enough sit-ups—it's the fat and fluid between your skin and your abdominal muscles that dictates whether or not you'll see muscle definition and that six-pack.

You may ask why there are no exercises for your abdominal muscles in this workout. There's a reason for that—they aren't necessary. And yet, most fighters still have incredible midsections. So what's their secret? When it comes to the techniques boxers use to prepare for a fight, everything emanates from their core, whether it's power, speed, or balance—that is their foundation. All roads lead to the core, so all roads lead out.

In this workout, you are consciously flexing your core muscles during every punch, turn of the rope, and bodyweight exercise, so your abs are always involved and remain engaged 100 percent of the time. It's a tactic that's necessary to improve the accuracy of your punches, making them faster and more precise. But it also helps to strengthen and define your abs, while the high-intensity pace of the program burns away the fat to reveal a sleeker, more defined midsection that's as efficient as it is impressive.

Sleekify Is Plateau-Proof

Your body is the perfect machine, designed to survive by adapting to many of the stresses life places on it. Do the same workout day after day, then, and your muscles quickly figure out an easier way to handle whatever demands you're placing on them using less effort and fewer calories. It's why most exercise routines hit a "plateau"—or, in other words, a place where the results simply stop, even though you continue to exercise week in and week out.

You're left with no choice but to figure out new ways to surprise your muscles, such as increasing the length or intensity of your workout regime, or lifting heavier weights. It's a process that takes a certain amount of creativity and exercise knowledge you may not have, but more important, it requires you to be ever vigilant about exactly when to modify your workout. Most of us aren't amateur kinesiologists, and as a result, even workouts that work eventually stop working.

Sleekify never reaches that point of no return, because it's impossible to master by design. All of the greatest fighters of all time may have excelled in certain areas of the sport, but none has ever excelled in every aspect of the sport. Not a single boxer who has ever stepped in the ring—from Jack Johnson to Floyd Mayweather—has ever truly mastered everything there is to know of boxing, which is what makes boxing such a beautiful thing to explore.

Through patience, repetition, and staying consistent with the program, you will never master but will always succeed with Sleekify, no matter how often you use it.

Sleekify Satisfies Your Spartan Soul

When was the last time you learned a skill that others envied? When was the last time you mastered something you couldn't wait to show off?

As adults, we never take on new things as often as we did when we were younger. We become set in our ways, following the same paths in life out of fear, or because we'd rather stay in our comfort zone. That lack of self-exploration leaves many people feeling unsatisfied. They never get a sense of gratification because they never feel as if they're completing anything new and exciting. This book will change that.

By learning Sleekify, you'll gain a sense of achievement that doesn't come from ordinary workouts. It's one of the few workouts that require your mind to be actively engaged right alongside your muscles. It kicks you out of your comfort zone and lets you experience that feeling of achievement that comes only with trying something new, something that's not easy to master—or in Sleekify's case, impossible to master—so you always feel good about yourself.

But what places Sleekify in an entirely different category is how it gives you a set of skills everyone around you wishes they could acquire. Not everyone is equally impressed with someone who can run marathons or ride a road bike for a hundred miles. But it's undeniable how both men and women alike admire the grace, speed, and strength that a boxer exudes when performing his or her craft. These are the abilities you will learn through Sleekify—abilities that make an impression not only on your physique, but on everyone who ever watches you perform what you're about to learn in this book.

Sleekify Exhausts You—Then Energizes You

One of the most common compliments I'm paid by my clients, no matter who they are or what they do in life, is that after they finish one of my workouts, they have an influx of energy that gets them through the day.

You want to have a powerful engine inside a Ferrari body. If you're all show and no go, if you build muscle and drop a few pounds but can't move your muscles through all planes of motion, you'll never enjoy the full quality of life that you could be having. With Sleekify, you can achieve a toned, highly defined body, but you'll also develop an engine inside that body that ensures it's a high-performance vehicle capable of doing anything—one that can pull off what it's advertising to do from the outside.

Sleekify Doesn't Follow Trends—It Sets Them

"New" training concepts such as interval training (where you vary the intensity of your cardio workout) and High-Intensity Interval Training (HIIT)—an advanced technique that combines quick, short bursts of high-intensity exercise with longer bursts of low-intensity exercise—are all the rage now.

That's because interval training has been shown to drastically improve stamina and speed, cause your body to use more fat as fuel, and even help build and preserve more lean muscle, compared to the "steady-state" approach to cardio—exercising at an even, unvarying moderate pace for a specific amount of time—that most people lean on.

But to be honest, they are just spin-offs of techniques boxers have been using for centuries. Sleekify is an interval-based routine that changes intensity throughout the program, designed to utilize stored glycogen—the stored carbohydrates your body turns to first when you begin exercising—at a rapid pace. The faster you can deplete your glycogen, the sooner your body can turn to its own stored body fat as a fuel source instead.

Sleekify Puts You—and Keeps You—in the Zone

And by "zone," I mean *all* of your fat-burning zones.

In order to improve your cardiovascular abilities and significantly burn fat, experts say you need to exercise hard enough to keep your heart rate within your target heart zone for twenty minutes or more.

To figure out your target heart zone, you just subtract your age from 220 to find your maximum heart rate (or MHR), then multiply that number by .65—this is your minimum training rate. Next, take your maximum heart rate again and multiply it by .8—this is your maximum training rate. The area between those two numbers is your target heart rate—or what some consider the "fat-burning zone."

There are other zones that produce different benefits. For example, to allow your muscles to recover, you could work out at a low-intensity zone (50 to 65 percent of your MHR). That's about a pace where you could talk as you exercise, but singing would be too difficult.

Or to improve your overall endurance and burn more calories, you could elevate your heart rate to between 80 and 85 percent of your MHR. To know if you've ever been in that zone, that's a tempo that usually makes it difficult to speak more than a few words without having to take a breath.

Finally, you could exercise in brief bursts at a high-intensity pace that reaches 90 to 95 percent of your MHR, which helps to increase your anaerobic threshold. Not only does this speed burn the most calories per minute, but it also increases the total amount of oxygen your body uses to recover after you're done exercising—so you burn additional calories for hours afterward.

Training in every zone possible can give your body a more well-rounded cardiovascular experience that produces maximum benefits. But trying to pull that off using a piece of cardio equipment requires breaking your stride constantly in order to push buttons to change the angle, speed, or resistance of the equipment you're using.

With Sleekify, there is no pressing or guessing. It's designed to take your heart rate through its paces—all of them—so you never have to worry about your workout.

Sleekify Is Excuse-Proof

Being able to exercise without equipment is extremely important, especially if you want to stay committed to an exercise plan. In order to say true long enough to a program so that you reap all of the results—and be able to maintain those results—it has to be able to fit into your day and become part of your lifestyle.

What puts Sleekify above most routines is that you can do it anywhere: in your home or apartment, on vacation, indoors or outdoors—basically anyplace you feel comfortable executing the Sleekify routine. It really doesn't require any excess equipment or space because instead of requiring fancy pieces of gym gear, Sleekify uses your body as the machine. In fact, your only investment beyond this book that you'll ever have to make is in a jump rope, a pair of light hand weights (not required), and a little bit of your time to break a sweat.

Enough talk: It's time to start Sleekifying!

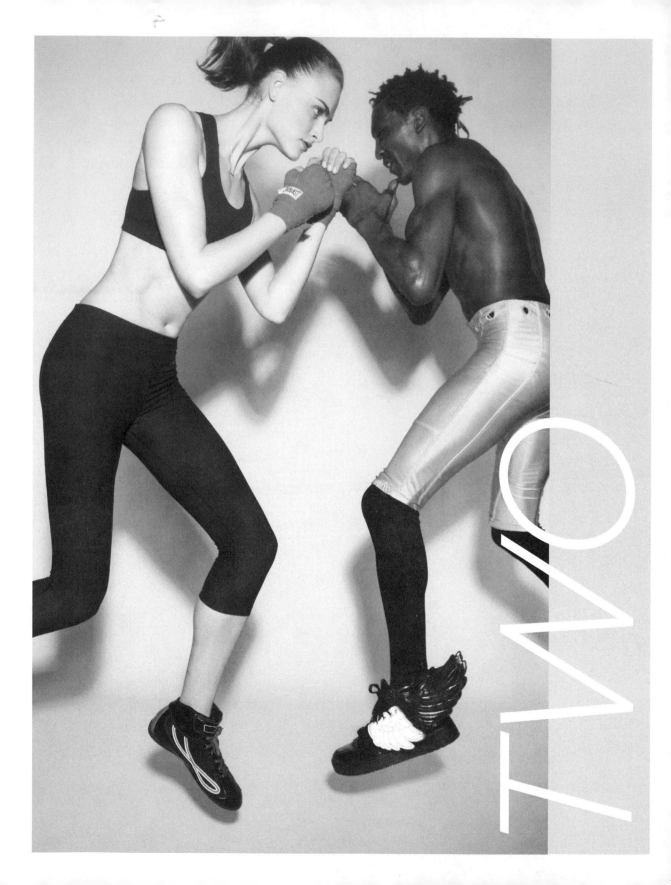

TWO

SLEEKIFY: YOUR BODY— THE EXERCISE EDGE

MY PHILOSOPHY ON WEIGHT LOSS—OR AS I LIKE TO CALL IT, MY "AERO-philosophy"—is simple.

In order for your body to become honed and sleek—to become leaner, stronger, fitter, and faster than you were yesterday—you need to commit to exercise, watch your diet, and bolster your mental fortitude. Without all three of these factors always in play, you will never Sleekify your body in a way that goes beyond whatever few and fleeting successes you may have experienced using conventional fat-burning programs in the past.

THE SLEEKIFY WORKOUT—EXPLAINED!

If you want to learn a different language, there's no faster way to do it than move to a country that speaks that language and totally immerse yourself in its culture. That same principle applies to fitness.

A body reflects whatever it does. If it's asked to lift larger, heavier weights at a slow pace, it will develop larger, heavier muscles. But if you put it in an atmosphere of doing quick, light, highly repetitive movements and keep it there, it will reflect that as well and allow you to develop a lighter, leaner, and faster physique. That's why cardio-based, light-weight drills and exercises—movements that are repeated over and over again at varying speeds for varied amounts of time—are the backbone of the Sleekify exercise plan and what all athletes known for their speed do in order to hone their bodies and reach their bodies' highest potential.

It's also why my clients come back from their checkups and brag to me about how their doctors are left scratching their heads when they come into their offices with the cardiovascular conditioning and resting heart rates of professional athletes. Their physicians may not understand why my clients are that healthy, and although it's always gratifying to hear them say that, it never surprises me. Through Sleekify, my clients experience incredible weight loss and an indescribable influx of energy. It's also why you will, too—and why Sleekify will have you looking like a world champion within a month.

THE BASICS OF THE WORKOUT

The Sleekify exercise program is an intense, full-body plan that utilizes as many muscle fibers as possible. It consumes more oxygen than the average cardio workout and creates a higher metabolic demand on your body. However, it's important that you pay attention to the basics and do it right, not only for safety's sake, but for the effectiveness of the workout—I want you to succeed 100 percent!

The entire program is divided into eight unique boxing-based workouts. You'll use each workout for a total of three days, then immediately move on to the next three-day workout in the schedule for the entire twenty-eight-day plan. Every six days, you'll give your body a rest by taking one day off.

(Does that sound like a lot of time? It's not, when you're talking just twenty-eight days for a workout that doesn't involve driving to the gym. But if you need to, you can modify this plan to fit your own time availability and commitment level. I describe how on page 21.)

In a nutshell, your schedule will look like this:

Days 1–3:	Workout A
Days 4–6:	Workout B
Day 7:	REST
Days 8–10:	Workout C
Days 11–13:	Workout D
Day 14:	REST
Days 15–17:	Workout E
Days 18–20:	Workout F
Day 21:	REST
Days 22–24:	Workout G
Days 25–27:	Workout H
Day 28:	REST

Each of the eight workouts is composed of a mix of three different types of boxing-based exercises and drills.

1. **AEROBOX®:** In every workout, you'll be practicing a series of shadowboxing drills that will have you throwing a variety of punches—the jab, the straight power punch, the double jab, the hook, and the uppercut—as well as a few defensive maneuvers that are meant to keep your body moving.

2. **AEROJUMP™:** You'll also be executing a variety of different jump rope exercises that will allow you to achieve maximum cardiovascular results in about one-third to one half the time of conventional cardio machines.

3. **AEROSCULPT™:** Finally, you'll be performing a mix of lower-body bodyweight exercises (no weights or machines required) that will improve your strength, balance, and coordination, as well as build lean, sleek muscle that will be hard to hide once the fat begins to disappear.

As you progress from week to week, you'll learn how to perform new exercises, punches, or drills. You'll also be reminded which past exercises, punches, or drills you'll be repeating (and should already be familiar with) from a previous chapter.

Unlike a typical workout program, where counting repetitions is the standard, with Sleekify:

- You'll count punches (which can range from throwing 32 up to 128).
- You'll count sets (which, when throwing certain combinations of punches, can range from repeating a combo of punches from 8 to 32 times).
- But most important, you'll count time. All of the Aerojump and Aerosculpt exercises—and some of the Aerobox moves—won't ask you to count reps. Instead, you'll do each for a certain number of seconds (which can range from 30 to 180 seconds).

PRE-SLEEKIFY YOURSELF

Before you start the Sleekify workout program, it absolutely pays off in the long run for your body to really understand the new demands that are going to be made of it and to practice—and perfect—a few key moves first. That way when you begin the program, you'll already have a level of experience with certain drills, so you'll feel less frustration and get more from every movement.

The Basics of Jumping Rope

There's a reason why jumping rope remains the cornerstone of every boxer's workout and has rapidly become one of the more preferred workouts for all athletes.

It helps you build and develop an aerobic foundation, requires minimal space, burns between 600 and 1,500 calories an hour (depending on your weight and the speed and intensity at which you're jumping), plus it works both your upper and lower body simultaneously. It's also one of the most effective ways to improve stamina, your foot and hand speed, agility, eye-foot-hand coordination, and your sense of balance simultaneously.

CUSTOMIZING THE SLEEKIFY PROGRAM TO YOUR LIFESTYLE

While the best results will come from following this program to its fullest, life has a way of upending our best-laid plans. Here's what I recommend:

Maximum Sleekify: To reap the most results from the program, it's my hope that you'll perform it—just as my clients do—to the letter, which means sticking to the twenty-eight-day program without adapting it in any way. Doing so will mean you'll be spending about forty-five to sixty minutes exercising six days a week (taking one day off after each week) for four straight weeks.

The more you do this program, the better it will be for your body. Remember, you want your body in a state of perpetual motion. That means you could even try doing this work-out—or some elements of this workout—twice a day, even if it is just performing the combinations and punches within the program at demo and exercise speed (which I'll explain later on in the book) when you wake up, and then executing the workout at fight speed (a pace I'll also explain later in the book) in the evening.

Minimum Sleekify: Even though the Sleekify program is convenient enough to do anywhere, I know that there will be times when you may not have as many minutes to invest.

If, on certain days, you simply do not have the forty-five to sixty minutes to devote to Sleekify, I would rather have you divide up the program into smaller portions than have you rush through it. Doing two smaller sessions of Sleekify—for example, performing two thirty-minute routines instead of one sixty-minute session—will still burn the same amount of total calories. In fact, splitting up the program temporarily revs your metabolism twice in the day instead of once, so your body burns through more calories after your workout.

If you have only a half hour to devote to your workout for the entire day, then cut the workout in half by doing half of the required repetitions, sets, and time. For example, if you're asked to do an Aerojump exercise for 180 seconds, do it for 90 instead. If you're told to repeat a combination of punches 32 times, then do it 16 instead.

Unlike many forms of cardio that may also challenge your body, strengthen your heart, and burn calories, jumping rope also gets your mind involved, giving you a deeper sense of accomplishment afterward because of the concentration, rhythm, and timing required. In other words, staying in place will help you go further.

Forget what you think you know

If you have any experience with jumping rope, you may need to unlearn what you may have learned in gym class. Jumping rope the right way isn't about jumping as high as you can, pulling your heels to your butt, and slamming your feet to the floor.

That type of jump—what most people call a "schoolgirl jump"—may have been okay when you were ten years old or weighed less than a hundred pounds. But when you're an adult—with a body that's no longer growing, is less resilient, and is a lot heavier— that style of jumping is a major problem because it's too abusive to your knees, shins, and feet.

Look at every misstep as a leap forward

For some people, the movement of jumping rope just comes naturally. For others, it may take a lot more work and time to get that rhythm down. But once you do get that rhythm down, it's a foundation that's yours for life—sort of like learning to ride a bike— and it will provide a platform that will allow you to build new challenging maneuvers and keep you jumping.

If that's you, then I need you to rethink how you approach working out. What a lot of people don't understand, and why a lot of people throw down the rope in frustration, is that nobody ever taught them how to jump rope, which, when done correctly, is a lot easier and simpler than it looks.

But I won't lie. Your body may feel confused and ask you "What hit me?" That's only because it's experiencing something that it's most likely never experienced before. You're finally taxing it in ways that you never taxed it before, in a way you can't achieve by running, cycling, doing step classes, or whatever aerobic activity you usually choose to use.

Last, remember that a rocket burns more fuel getting off the ground than it does when it's airborne. What that means is this: When you're learning something new, you exert more effort throughout the process, which means you'll burn more calories. Each time you perform a new, challenging maneuver in my workout, you will be repeating that effort, and subsequently, burning even more calories. So when you trip up—and you will trip up, because I've been jumping rope for thirty-five years and I still trip up—laugh it off, and remember why you're jumping in the first place. You're learning to fly, so don't let anything stop you from your goal and have the fortitude to continue.

With jumping rope—and the rest of the exercises in the program—it's all about patience and repetition. Just putting in the effort—even if you lack coordination, speed, and strength to start—will create results. The only way you'll never see results is by quitting before you conquer.

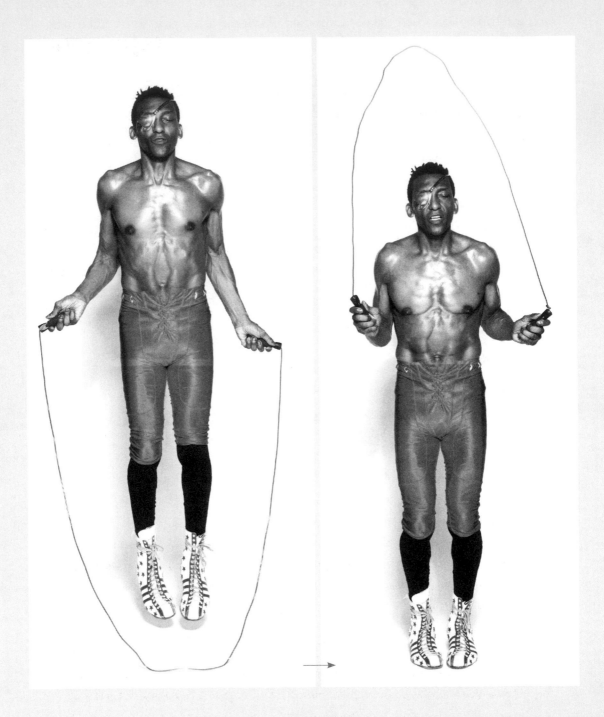

BASIC JUMP

(This beginner exercise works on your timing and coordination, which will help you master the other variations in the program.)

START POSITION: Start by holding the rope at both ends—your arms should be down at your sides at waist level, palms facing the ceiling. Step forward so that the middle of the rope is right behind your heels.

THE MOVE: Keeping your hands close to your body, begin turning the rope forward, rotating only from your wrists. Once the rope comes down toward your feet, take a tiny hop—no more than an inch or so—to allow the rope to pass underneath you. Land on the balls of your feet—not flat-footed or on your heels (in fact, your heels should never touch the floor)—and repeat at a pace of roughly 132 rotations per minute.

Head-to-Toe Aero-Tips

- Eyes: You may look down at first, but try to keep your eyes looking forward, not staring down at your feet, which can strain your neck. If you have the option to jump in front of the mirror, do it, but if you don't, you'll see the rope coming down in front of you as it turns. As you see the rope come down past your eyes, jump the rope. Try to track the movement of the rope—it may be hard to do at first because it's not in your instincts to do so, but you'll start picking it up as you practice. Remember this: See the rope—jump the rope. It's all about the timing.

- Arms: Keep your arms bent at the elbow at about a 90-degree angle, but concentrate on tucking your elbows in close to your sides. Bringing your hands, elbows, and arms up to shoulder level makes your shoulders do the brunt of the work (and will tire them out before the rest of your body gets a good sweat).

   Raising your hands also shortens the height of the rope, which you don't want to do—the shorter the rope, the higher you'll have to jump off the floor in order to let it pass underneath you. Not only can you hurt your feet, shins, and hips, but this will throw you into the anaerobic zone immediately and make jumping rope feel like you're running a series of sprints without the benefit of a warm-up. It's like trying to do a series of high hurdles back to back to back—it's brutal to your body and within just a few jumps, you'll feel like you can't do any more.

- Hands: Keep your hands at waist level the entire time—the higher you raise your hands, the shorter the rope becomes and you'll be more likely to stumble.

    Also, your wrists should be what make the rope go, so try to remember that your wrists are the motors that get the rope turning the entire time.

    One thing I have to watch out for with clients is having their dominant side affect their jumps. If you're right-handed, that means you're most likely going to be "right-side dominant," which causes many people to rely more on their right side—hands, arms, legs, etc.—rather than split the workload evenly with their left side.

    That means as you jump, you might forget to turn your left wrist, placing most of the work on your right wrist. That's okay at the start, since you may just want to get airborne, but just be cautious of that and try to turn your left hand in time with your right—and vice versa if you're left-handed.

- Legs: Always keep your legs and feet together throughout the move (unless asked to do otherwise in some of the other advanced jumps in the program). Your legs act as rockets that propel you off the ground when you jump up, and conversely as shock absorbers when you land, so most of the energy from every hop is absorbed throughout your calves, quadriceps, and glutes.

    I remind clients to think about a ballet dancer or basketball player as they rise up, keep their legs together, then land on the toes, then shift their bodyweight down to the balls of their feet—it should feel like one continuous, fluid motion.

- Heels: Keep your heels up off the floor the entire time—you never land or take off from your heels at any point.

- Pace: Your hands, not your feet, control the pace. Your feet react to the pace of your hands.

BEFORE YOU TAKE YOUR FIRST JUMP . . .
MASTER THE PACE

Although as a starting pace, I like people to turn the rope about 132 times in sixty seconds, I'm not expecting you to count the entire time. Instead, it's more about getting a feel for that pace and knowing what 132 rotations a minute feels like.

First thing to know: 132 rotations may sound like a lot, but your hands have the potential to move that fast—in fact, most people's hands are generally faster than their legs. This drill—which I prefer clients use before they even begin attempting the basic jump—helps get the right muscles in your forearms to fire and gives your hands a sense of how fast they need to move in order to match that pace perfectly.

This drill can help cut back some of the frustration of learning how to jump, which—and be ready for it to happen—is going to happen to you because it happens to everybody. In fact, it still happens to me.

The trick: Take both handles of the jump rope in one hand—preferably your dominant hand to start—and let the rope hang down by your side. Then, without jumping, start turning the rope using only the wrist with your elbow close to your body. The rope should look almost like a propeller blade, spinning along the side of your body.

You can use a timer—or just count it out—but try to see how many rotations you can do in one minute with each hand. As you get comfortable with the pace, you can even try jumping at the same time to help work on your timing before you actually begin to hop over the rope.

If you're truly serious about this program to help reveal your body's true potential, this is something you'll practice every day—even on days you don't have to exercise. I want you to think of it as the runway to a higher level of fitness. The more you do it, the more skilled you'll become at jumping rope, and trust me, it will more than pay off in the end.

EVERYTHING NECESSARY TO
SUCCESSFULLY SLEEKIFY!

The beauty of Sleekify is that the biggest investment you'll ever make is your time. Here are the only things you'll need to get started:

Supportive footwear: Wear a pair of running shoes or cross-trainers to ensure your feet stay shock-protected and stable as you jump. They will also give you the grip you'll need when throwing punches and performing many of the Aerosculpt exercises. If you're not in the market for a new pair of shoes, then you can get away with buying a pair of gel shoe inserts for under the ball of the foot to help absorb impact.

A forgiving surface: The only area you'll need to Sleekify is a four-foot square—but what's below you matters. Avoid concrete, macadam, or other hard surfaces that don't have much give. Instead, opt for springier surfaces that are easier on the joints, such as hardwood floors, a blacktop driveway, or even low-cut carpeting.

A jump rope: What I particularly recommend is a PVC rope with a ball-bearing handle like the AeroSpace Rainmaker (the one I have my clients use). The reason it's my top choice is that you'll get an instant response from the rope as you twirl it—the moment you flick your wrists, the rope turns for you. The Rainmaker also keeps an even arc as you spin it, so there's always a big loop to jump through—a plus that helps prevent frustrating tangles and eases your learning curve.

Stay away from beaded varieties and weighted ropes, which can compromise your form and increase your risk of injury initially. Weighted ropes also thrust you into an anaerobic zone, which can cause your body to work much harder than it's prepared to do. Also, watch out for ropes made from a material that's too light. If the rope's too flimsy, it will slow down as it rotates, causing you to jump higher and put more stress on your knees in order to jump over it.

Light hand weights (optional): To get more results each time you punch, I encourage my clients to invest in a pair of lightweight dumbbells (one to three pounds maximum) that they can hold in each hand. However, I would avoid using them until you truly feel comfortable and have your form down with each Aerobox exercise. And even then, I highly recommend using hand weights performing punches at only demo and exercise speeds—never fight speed.

THE BASICS OF THROWING A PUNCH

About two-thirds of the Sleekify workout routine is an upper-body cardio experience, so it engages your entire body in a way that it's not used to. That means every muscle gets involved from head to toe, so your body burns the maximum amount of calories in minimum time. Plus, because your upper body (arms) can generally move faster than your lower body (legs), it allows you to experience a more intense workout than ever before. That's what makes the Aerobox sections—the portions of the workout that require you to perform short bursts of shadowboxing—so vital to the program.

Throw with your body—not your arms

Many people think that when you punch, it's all about your arms and nothing more. Not true. When you punch correctly, you're using your legs and your core muscles just as much as your arms. In fact, your arms are merely where all of your energy gets released. But it begins and builds from your foundation, which are your core and leg muscles.

Punching is all about transferring your energy/weight forward along a specific plane or pathway. If all you use are your arms to punch when using the program, it's far less taxing because you'll use fewer muscles and burn far fewer calories. But if you learn how to throw every punch properly—when you understand how to turn your body in sync with each punch, when you can feel your feet gripping the floor so you can drive that power through your core muscles and out through each fist—that's when you'll see the most benefits.

Find your own performance zone

It's important to realize that although the pacing of Sleekify may be different than training at a real gym, the boxing techniques you'll be performing are no different than what you would be expected to pull off at a real fight gym by the world's best boxing trainers.

How fast you throw each punch is extremely important. Although you don't have to be as fast as the next person, like I will continually say throughout this book, the benefit is in the effort. All you need to do is try your hardest and you will benefit the same way as someone faster. It's about finding your personal high-performance zone.

That said, each time you punch, you'll be asked to try to throw them at a specific speed. Here are the three speeds you'll be expected to maintain when executing any punch or combination of punches:

DEMO SPEED: Demo speed (which you'll see in the charts as DS) is the slowest and most basic of the tempos. Basically, each punch that you throw should take two seconds—one second for the punch to go out and one second to pull your fist back into the starting position.

Why you'll be using this tempo is easy—it's a great way to prepare your mind and muscles for what you're about to ask of them. That way, your form should be perfect once you're ready to perform the same punches at a quicker speed. As you become fitter following the program, you'll also become more proficient at throwing each punch and combo of punches, so you'll notice you won't be required to throw as many punches at this speed later in the routine.

NOTE: Once you feel comfortable throwing punches, you can begin holding a pair of hand weights while performing any punch or punch combo at this speed.

EXERCISE SPEED: Exercise speed (which you'll see in the charts as ES) is twice as fast as demo speed. You'll know you have the pacing down if each punch that you throw takes one second—that means about ½ second for the punch to go out and about ½ second to pull your fist back in.

NOTE: Just like demo speed, as you learn each punch, you may also use hand weights while performing any punch or punch combo at this speed.

FIGHT SPEED: Fight speed (which you'll see in the charts as FS) is the fastest (and highest-intensity) of the tempos. To do it right, you have to move about twice as fast as exercise speed, so be ready to move as quickly as possible. That means each punch should take about ½ second—¼ second for the punch to go out; ¼ second for the punch to come in.

NOTE: Fight speed is extremely fast, which makes using hand weights out of the question.

Finally—and listen closely, because this is probably the most important key to being successful at the Aerobox sections of the Sleekify workout—you *must* try to always fully execute every punch and move, even at the elevated speeds. Do not try to abbreviate the drills in any way—the more you can keep form as you switch up to the higher speeds, the bigger the benefit your body can expect. Will it be hard? Yes, but that's where the treasure's buried.

THE STANCES TO EXPECT

Anytime you'll be asked to throw a punch, it will be from one of three stances—Pyramid, Orthodox, or Southpaw.

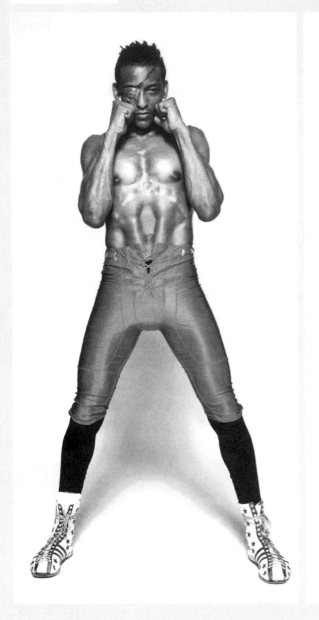
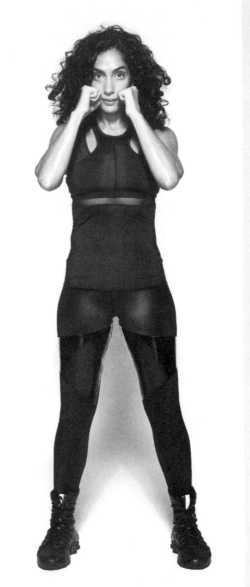

This stance is a little bit of a departure from boxing because it's not a traditional fighting stance. Instead, the Pyramid is more of a martial arts stance I use with clients for several reasons. One, I like to have them focus on the technique of their punches and not worry about all of the complexities of where their feet should be and if they're balanced properly. This position makes it easier to focus on one thing at a time, which in this case is punching properly. And two, I like them to be ambidextrous and be able to throw punches with either fist. This stance lets them do both with ease.

THE POSITION: Stand straight with your feet slightly wider than shoulder width apart. Bring your fists up along the sides of your face (about an inch away from it) and position them right below your cheekbones. Your palms should be facing in toward each other with your knuckles pointing toward the ceiling.

Aero-Tips

- Legs: Your knees should be slightly bent—muscles tense—with your bodyweight evenly distributed on both feet.
- Head: Keep your head and neck in line with your back and look straight ahead—don't arch your neck forward, but let your chin drop down slightly.
- Feet: The toes of both feet should be facing forward.
- Arms: Your elbows should be slightly out to your sides and not directly below your fists.

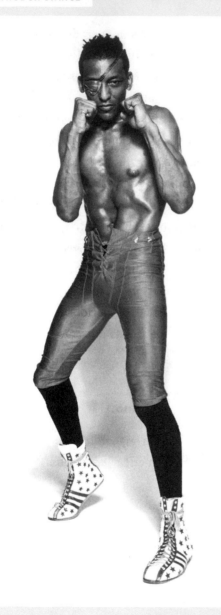

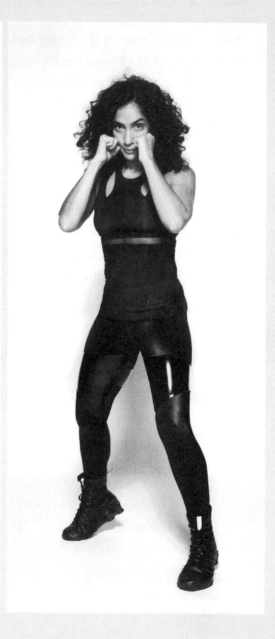

This left foot forward, right foot back stance is what orthodox boxers (right-handed fighters like me) rely on. The position keeps your left fist and left leg closer to your opponent, leaving your back hand—your right fist—farther back so you get the weight of your body behind the punch.

To get into the stance, take a half step forward with your left foot and keep your toes pointing straight ahead. Next, take a half step back with your right foot and turn it at a 45-degree angle so that your toes are pointing away from your body. Imagine you're standing in the center of a clock—you'll know your feet are positioned perfectly if your left foot points to twelve and your right foot is pointing between two and three o'clock.

Twist slightly at the waist to the right (boxers do this to give their opponents less surface to hit, while it also allows for more power in the punch from the right side). Finally, bring your fists up along the sides of your face (palms facing in and knuckles pointing toward the ceiling) and you're ready to go.

Aero-Tips

- Legs: Just like the Pyramid stance, your knees should be slightly bent—muscles semi-tense—with your bodyweight evenly distributed on both feet.
- Arms: Just like the Pyramid stance, your elbows should remain slightly out to your sides and not directly below your fists.
- Feet: You want to be on the ball of your right foot with your left foot flat on the floor—feet shoulder width apart. For now, your back foot should never be flat on the floor at any time. Meanwhile, your lead foot should be like the needle of the compass, always pointing the direction you want to travel—in this case, toward the shadow opponent in front of you.

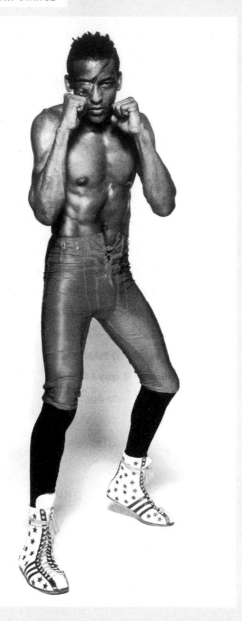
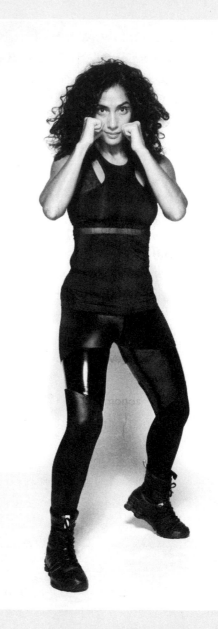

This right foot forward, left foot back stance—used by left-handed boxers—is the exact opposite position of Orthodox, but it serves the same purpose. It keeps your right fist and right leg in closer to your opponent, so your back hand—in this case, your left fist—is the big threat.

The stance is easy to get into if you've already mastered Orthodox—that's because it's the same position, only in reverse! To do it properly, take a half step forward with your right foot (keeping your toes pointing straight ahead), then take a half step back with your left foot and turn it 45 degrees so that your toes are pointing away from your body. Remember that clock? This time, your left toes should point between nine and ten o'clock.

Twist slightly at the waist to the left (to give your imaginary opponent less surface to hit and to add power when throwing from your left side). Finally, bring your fists up along the sides of your face (palms facing in and knuckles pointing toward the ceiling).

Aero-Tips

- Legs: Just like the Pyramid stance, your knees should be slightly bent—muscles tense—with your bodyweight evenly distributed on both feet.
- Arms: Just like the Pyramid stance, your elbows should remain slightly out to your sides and not directly below your fists.
- Feet: You want to be on the ball of your left foot with your right foot flat on the floor—feet shoulder width apart. For now, your back foot should never be flat on the floor at any time.

THE PUNCHES TO EXPECT

Now that you know how to position your body to throw a punch, it's time to learn how to do exactly that. For the purposes of Sleekify, here are the only punches you need to know:

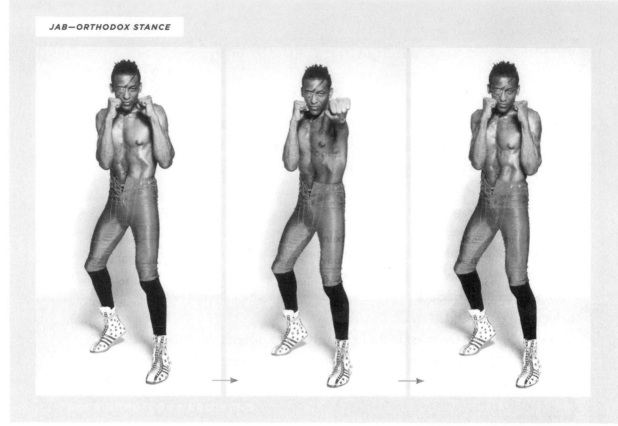

JAB

The jab is the most versatile—and the most commonly used—punch in boxing. It may not be a knockout blow, but in my sport, it's the workhorse that does everything from scoring points and setting up more powerful blows to keeping an opponent at a safe distance. In this program, however, it's the fastest of the punches, so throwing a lot of them consecutively—or mixing them into more advanced combinations—will quickly get your heart pumping and your upper body sculpted and Sleekified.

This basic punch comes from the lead side of your body (in other words, whichever foot is forward). For example, if your left foot is forward (Orthodox stance) and you throw a straight punch with your left hand, that's a jab—vice versa with your right side. So how can you do it perfectly for the purposes of my Sleekify program?

Like this:

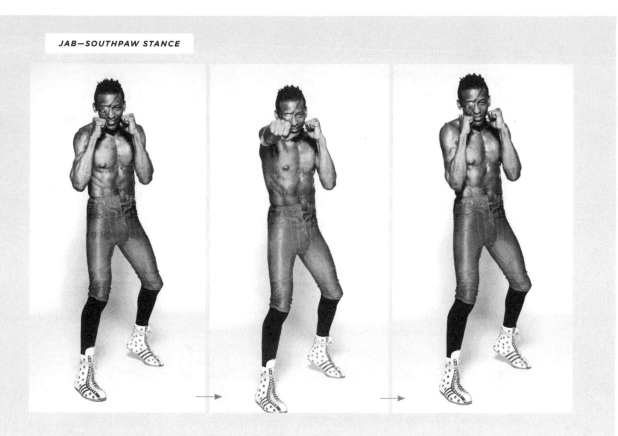

THE MOVE: Without moving your legs—and without turning your waist—throw your leading arm forward in a straight line from your face. As you punch, rotate your fist inward so that your palm ends up facing down toward the floor. Immediately bring your fist back in a straight line to the side of your face, rotating your arm outward as you go so that your fist ends up back in the starting position.

Aero-Tips

- Arm: You want to extend your arm as far as you can without locking your elbow. So if straightening your arm to the point of locking it is 100 percent, aim for extending your arm about 98 percent of the way.
- Elbow: The most common mistake people make is that they lift their elbow up before they throw the punch. This prevents you from getting as much power because you're

strictly using your biceps and triceps to move your arm—instead of your bi's, tri's, chest, shoulders, and forearms.

- Hand: Tighten your fist at the moment your arm is completely extended. When it's not "striking" an imaginary target in front of you, keep your hand in a fist, but relaxed until the next jab. Your opposite hand—whichever fist you're not throwing—should never leave the side of your face.

- Feet: Although your body will slightly project forward as you punch, at this point don't step forward or backward to try to pull back and make each punch more powerful—that's actually a different punch you'll learn later. There's really no torque of the body with the basic jab—all of the movement (and power) comes from your arm.

- Visualize this: Have you ever seen a moving piston inside its chamber? It travels exactly the same route back that it does moving forward—and at the same speed. That's how your arm should move, just like a piston, traveling straight and at the same speed, both going forward and coming back.

- And visualize this: Picture hitting an imaginary opponent directly in front of you with the knuckle of your middle finger. In order for that to happen, your wrist has to turn so your palm is facing the floor at the point of contact.

WAIT! HOW DO I DO IT FROM A PYRAMID STANCE? No problem. Even though this position prevents you from having a leading foot, you can still throw the punch exactly as described if your feet are even.

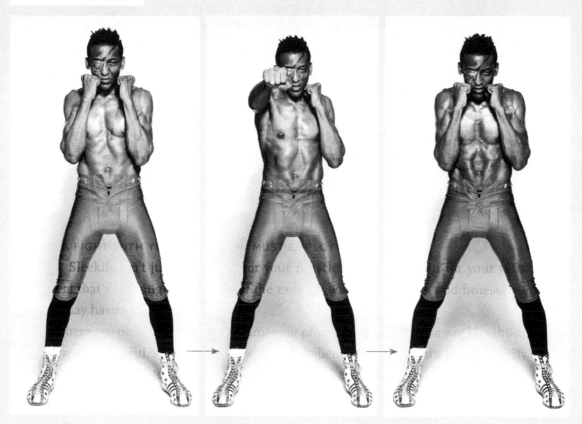

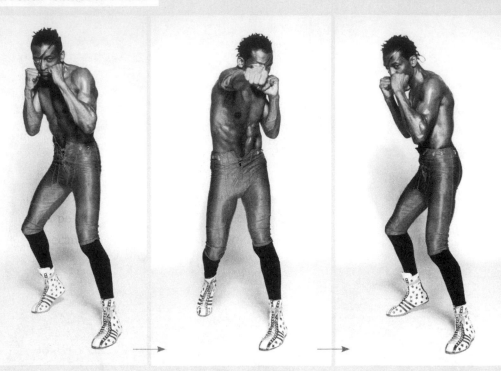

STRAIGHT POWER PUNCH

This full-body punch uses all of the muscles throughout your legs, hips, and core. Against an opponent, it's a threat because all those muscles working together allow you to generate a lot of power through your punch.

All that involvement takes energy, which is why many boxers—especially heavyweights—use it sparingly in a fight. But when it comes to reaching your goals even faster, this stronger punch burns a lot more calories, so consider it a threat that will help you knock out—and off—your unwanted body fat.

This basic punch comes from whichever fist is behind your body. For example, if your left foot is forward (Orthodox stance) and you throw a straight punch with your right hand, that's a power punch (or power right). If your right foot is forward (South-paw stance) and you throw a straight punch with your left hand, that's also a power punch (or power left).

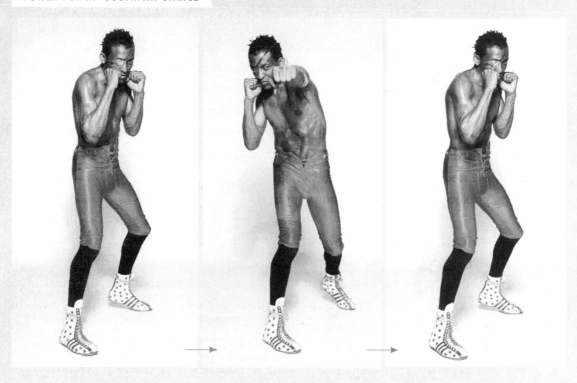

THE MOVE:

1.   Using whichever fist is farthest from your opponent, throw your arm forward in a straight line from your face, rotating your arm inward so that your palm ends up down once your arm is extended.

2.   As you throw the punch, simultaneously lift your back heel off the floor and pivot your back ankle outward as if you were squashing out a cigarette—keeping the ball of your back foot in place—and rotate your hips and shoulders into the punch.

3.   Reverse the motion by immediately bringing your fist back in a straight line to the side of your face (rotating your arm outward as you go) while simultaneously pivoting your hips and shoulders back into the start position, lowering your back heel onto the floor.

- Hand: Just like the regular jab, tighten your fist at the moment your arm is completely extended, then keep it relaxed (but still in a fist) the rest of the time. Your opposite hand—whichever fist you're not throwing—should never leave the side of your face.
- Core: Keep your abs tight throughout the punch. Having them contracted helps with focus and control; plus it improves your ability to coordinate all of your muscles simultaneously.

WAIT! HOW DO I DO IT FROM A PYRAMID STANCE? In my workout, there will be times when you're throwing either a power left or right—and sometimes, alternating back and forth between the two for a series of punches.

When you throw your left hand, your right shoulder will naturally fall back, which automatically positions your right fist to be farther back and ready to deliver a power punch (and vice versa when throwing a right punch).

So even though you may start with your shoulders even with each other, once you throw the first punch in whatever combination of punches I ask you to do, your body will naturally angle itself so that you're able to rotate and deliver a power punch with either hand from this stance. Remember, engage the core: The hawk will fall from its perch if its feet aren't gripping the branch.

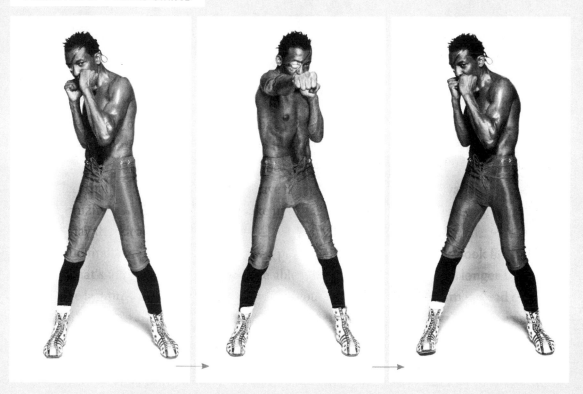

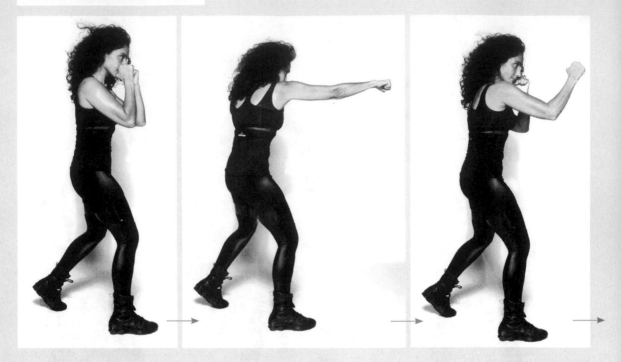

DOUBLE JAB

The double jab is exactly what it sounds like. It's two jabs thrown one after another by the same fist—and an effective way of bringing the intensity of the Sleekify program to a higher level.

THE MOVE:

1. Without moving your legs—and without turning your waist or shoulders—throw your leading arm forward in a straight line from your face.

2. As you punch, rotate your fist inward so that your palm ends up facing down toward the floor once your arm is fully extended. Immediately bring your fist halfway

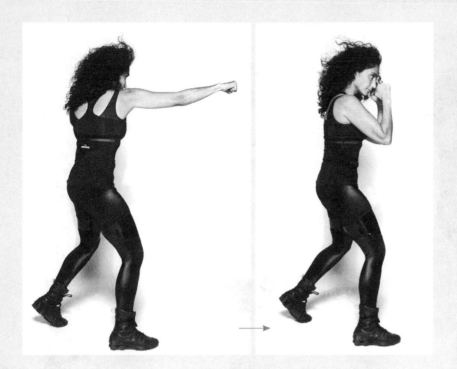

back in a straight line, rotating your arm outward as you go, then immediately extend a second jab forward using the same arm.

3.   Finally, quickly bring your fist in a straight line back to the side of your face so that your fist ends up in the starting position.

Aero-Tips

(The same tips that apply to a regular jab apply to the double jab, with just one change.)

- Arm: With the first jab, you want to extend your arm as far as you can without locking your elbow. With the second jab, you'll retract your arm only about 50 percent, but still rotate your fist as if you were throwing a full jab. Don't just push your fist

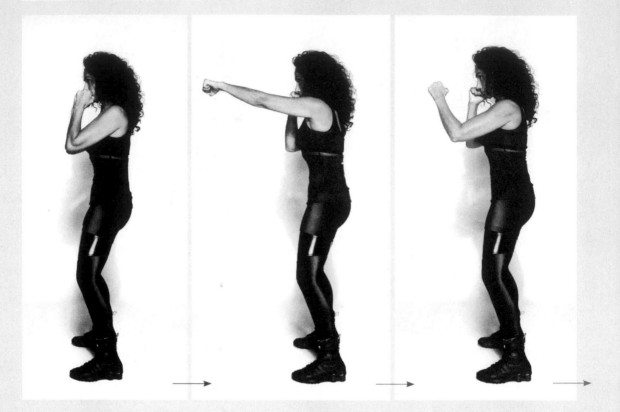

forward—instead, continue to rotate as you go and don't worry if your palm doesn't end facing the floor.

- Hand: Just like the regular jab, tighten your fist as your arm is extending, then keep it relaxed (but still in a fist) the rest of the time. Your opposite hand—whichever fist you're not throwing—should never leave the side of your face.

- Feet: Again, don't step forward or backward to try to pull back and make each punch more powerful—just allow your arm to do all the work.

- Visualize this: Imagine a woodpecker drilling into a tree. The jab is a highly repetitive

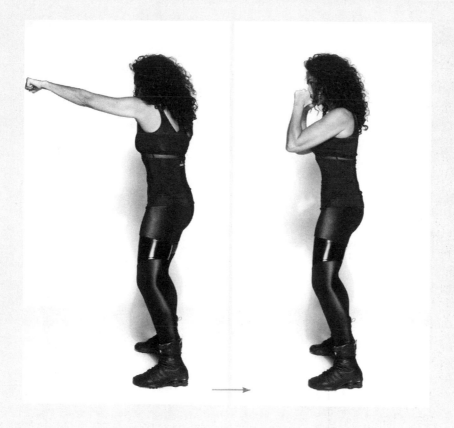

and focused quick punch designed to do damage through quick repetition rather than one powerful stroke.

WAIT! HOW DO I DO IT FROM A PYRAMID STANCE? Just like the regular jab, even though this position prevents you from having a leading foot, you can still throw the punch exactly as described.

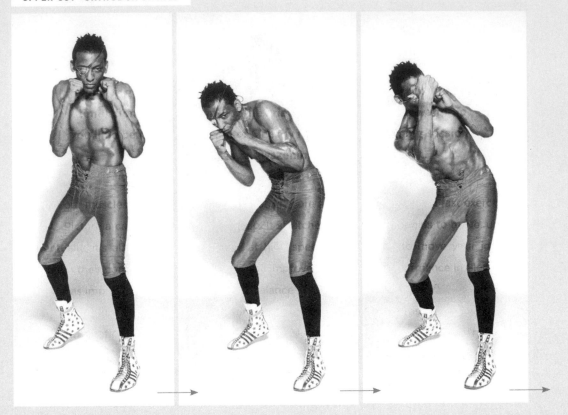

UPPERCUT

This devastating knockout punch—used when close to an opponent as a sneak attack that can slip between an opponent's defenses and land square on their chin—is one of the most powerful punches in any boxer's arsenal and can be thrown with either hand, no matter what stance you're in. But for fitness purposes, it tones your upper back, biceps, and obliques. It also adds variety to your punches, which will challenge your mind and allow you to pull off greater punching combinations that will tone your upper body and burn calories at a higher rate.

The uppercut is an upward-arcing punch not unlike a golf swing, but it takes a lot of effort to do it correctly. Dexterity is a key ingredient in being a successful fighter as well

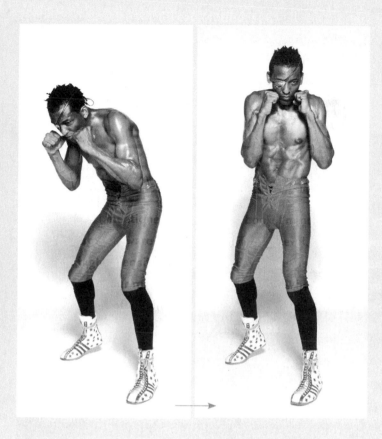

as being successful at this program. For you, all the effort required for performing an uppercut means utilizing even more muscles—and burning extra calories. It doesn't just knock down or surprise your opponent. It drops whatever unwanted fat is covering up your muscles as well.

THE MOVE:

To throw a regular uppercut, which uses the fist farther from your opponent (if you were standing in an Orthodox stance, that would be your right fist; if standing in South-paw stance, that would be your left fist):

1.   With your shoulders hunched slightly forward, bend your knees so that your body dips down about 3 to 4 inches, keeping your fists in close to your face.

2.   Begin to drop your back fist as you simultaneously swing upward (like a pendu-

lum) and outward so that as it leaves the side of your face, the palm of your fist ends up facing you, knuckles pointing at the ceiling on the upswing.

3.   Simultaneously transfer your bodyweight onto your back leg and begin pivoting off the ball of your back foot. As you go, quickly twist your hips and shoulders inward—this will line up your fist directly where you want it to be (about waist level, straight below your opponent's head) as you drive your fist upward—imagine you're aiming directly underneath an opponent's chin. At the point of impact, your elbow should be out and away, in front of your body.

4.   Reverse the motion by bringing your fist back toward your face as you rotate back into the starting position.

To throw a lead-side uppercut, which uses the fist closer to your opponent (if you were standing in an Orthodox stance, that would be your left fist; if standing in Southpaw stance, that would be your right fist):

1.   Tilt your body to the side of your leading hand (the hand you're going to punch with) so that your body isn't positioned perfectly straight up and down.

2.   Bend your knees so that your body dips down about 3 to 4 inches as you simultaneously twist your lead shoulder back, keeping your fists in close to your face.

3.   Begin to drop your front fist as you simultaneously swing upward (like a pendulum) and outward so that as it leaves the side of your face, the palm of your fist ends up facing you, knuckles pointing at the ceiling on the upswing. Your elbow should leave the body as you go.

4.   Simultaneously transfer your bodyweight onto your back leg and slightly pivot off the ball of your back foot. As you go, simultaneously twist your hips and shoulders inward—this will line up your fist directly where you want it to be (about waist level, straight below your opponent's head) as your fist arcs upward—imagine you're aiming directly underneath an opponent's chin.

5.   Reverse the motion by bringing your fist back toward your face as you rotate back into the starting position.

Aero-Tips

- Stop your fist about head height—going farther than that will slow down your pace, while punching too low will prevent you from challenging as many muscles and give you less of a workout.

- Legs: Don't forget to bend your knees—you want to flex and fire your leg muscles at the same time as you punch. Some of the power comes from your legs with this punch (with the rest coming from your core), so if you don't bend your knees, you'll never target those muscle fibers and won't get the most out of the exercise.

- Hips: Concentrate on keeping your hips low, which helps ground you as you punch. If your hips rise, you're trying to "jump" through the punch, instead of letting the rotation of your hips generate all the power.

- Hand: Tighten your fist at the very end of the punch, then keep it relaxed (but still in a fist) the rest of the time. Your opposite hand—whichever fist you're not throwing—should never leave the side of your face.

- Elbow: When you throw the uppercut, extend your arm so that your elbow is away from your body. Many people keep their elbows in close, which will limit your range of motion and give you less of a workout.

- Whether you're throwing a right or left uppercut, always tilt your body to the side the punch is coming from, so that your shoulder, fist, hip, and upper back turn into the punch at the same time.

WAIT! HOW DO I DO IT FROM A PYRAMID STANCE? Anytime I ask you to do the uppercut from this position, don't worry about pivoting off your foot—in fact, don't worry about your legs at all. I still want you to bend your knees, flex the muscles in your legs, and twist as you punch, but strictly focus on your core and upper body.

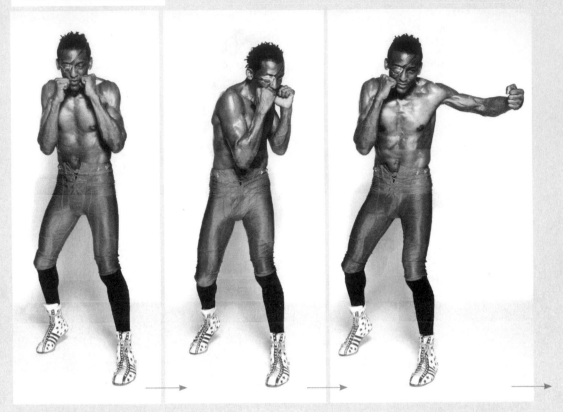

HOOK

The hook is another punch that opponents hate because it seems to come out of no-where. That's because their focus is dead ahead and the hook comes from the periphery. Often as a boxer, you don't pick it up until it's too late, since the fist swings in from the side instead of being thrown in a straight line, making it harder to defend against.

Here's how you do it:

THE MOVE:

To throw a regular hook, which uses the fist closer to your opponent (if standing in an Orthodox stance, that would be your left fist; if standing in Southpaw stance, that would be your right fist):

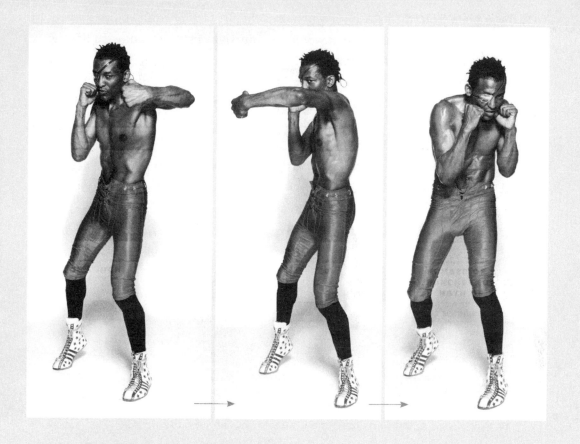

1.　Keeping your fists along the sides of your face, load up your punch by twisting from the waist and turning your lead shoulder—and the entire side of your upper body—back away from your imaginary opponent. Try to imagine an archer as they pull back the string of their bow.

2.　Release the punch by twisting your body forward, turning your hips into the punch as you pivot on the ball of your front foot.

3.　As you twist, simultaneously raise your elbow up as you move your fist away from your face and rotate it so that your palm faces you, thumb facing the ceiling. After the punch, your fist should end up about a foot from your face, with your shoulder, elbow, and fist all at the same height directly in front of your nose.

4.　Reverse the motion by simultaneously twisting your hips and bringing your arm and fist back through the same plane of motion to the starting position.

To throw a hook from the back foot, which uses the fist farther from your opponent (if standing in an Orthodox stance, that would be your right fist; if standing in Southpaw stance, that would be your left fist):

NOTE: This variation isn't a very commonly thrown punch, but it's still effective when used correctly—and ideal for adding more core strength into your workout. Because you throw the punch from your back side—the shoulder farther from your imaginary opponent—your arm will already be loaded back.

1.   Keeping your bodyweight evenly distributed between both feet, twist your body forward, turning your hips into the punch as you pivot on the ball of your front foot.

2.   As you twist, raise your elbow up as you move your fist away from your face and rotate it so that your palm faces you, thumb facing the ceiling. Your fist should end up about a foot from your face, with your shoulder, elbow, and fist all at the same height directly in front of your nose.

3.   Reverse the motion by twisting your hips and bringing your arm and fist back through the same plane of motion to the starting position.

Aero-Tips

- You want to make a circular motion with your fist—it should feel like if you continued to punch, your arm would draw a circle around your entire body.
- As you twist your shoulder back home, your whole arm should come back and your elbow returns to the side of your body.
- To get into the groove of it, imagine you're chopping tall stems of wheat with a scythe.
- Hands: The fist you're throwing should not leave the side of your face until your shoulder begins its rotation forward. Your opposite hand—whichever fist you're not throwing—should never leave the side of your face.

WAIT! HOW DO I DO IT FROM A PYRAMID STANCE? Even though both feet are parallel to each other in the Pyramid position, don't worry about pivoting your feet, since any foot movement will be ever so slight when punching for speed and in combination. You'll still get a surprising amount of explosive power when you throw the punch from this stance. And the better you get at it, the stronger and sleeker your midsection will become.

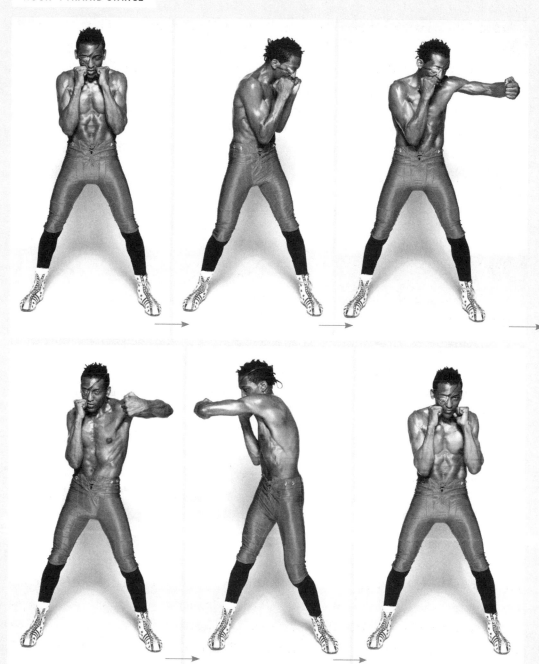

The hook can be the most difficult punch for people to learn because it's not as much of a natural movement as the other punches. To pull it off, you have to raise your elbow up as you twist forward so that your elbow, shoulder, and fist are all in a straight line by the time you've executed the punch, but the timing of this sometimes takes a lot more coordination than many people have.

That's why—for the purposes of my exercise program—I found a way to teach the hook that not only makes it easier to coordinate, but really works the abdominal and oblique muscles at the same time. My technique has you bring your arm up into the finished position—the impact position—before you even throw the punch, then lock your arm in place *before* twisting at the waist to put power into the punch.

Here's how you can practice it:

THE MOVE:

1.   Keeping your bodyweight centered between both feet, raise the elbow of your leading hand out to the side. Turn your wrist so that the palm of your fist is facing you, thumb facing the ceiling—your shoulder, elbow, and fist should all be at the same height directly in front of your nose (your fist about a foot from your face).

2.   Now lock that arm in place—from this point, you won't be bending it or straightening it, but keeping it fixed so that it moves with your body, not independently of it.

3.   Twisting from the waist, turn your shoulder and the entire side of your body back, then swing your arm forward as you turn your hips into the punch and pivot on the ball of your front foot. Don't drop your elbow or try to throw your fist—instead, let your body pull your arm around so the movement relies on your obliques, your abs, and your hip flexors.

4.   Reverse the motion by twisting your hips and bringing your arm and fist back through the same plane of motion to the starting position.

AERO-TIP—One quick way to know if you're throwing each punch properly is to use your elbow as your guide. At the end of every jab or power punch, your elbow should be straight; at the end of every uppercut, your elbow should be pointing straight down; at the end of every hook, your elbow should be pointing out in front of you.

AERO-TIP—Anytime you're eager to see results fast, you're more likely to cheat, whether you're conscious of it or not, by altering your posture to make a specific exercise, punch, or drill easier to perform. Instead of trusting what you may see in the mirror, try recording yourself performing your Aerobox, Aerojump, and Aerosculpt moves from several different angles—particularly from the side and back. It could reveal where you might be robbing yourself of results.

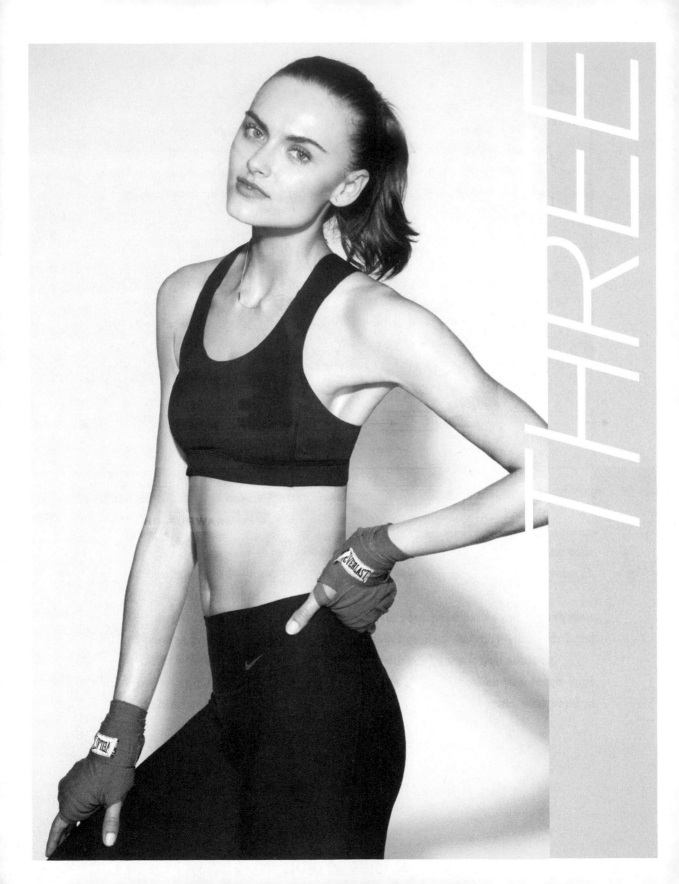

SLEEKIFY:
YOUR DIET—
THE NUTRITIONAL
EDGE

EVEN THOUGH YOU'LL SEE REMARKABLE WEIGHT LOSS RESULTS BY SIMPLY FOLLOWING the exercise portion of Sleekify, weight loss—like I mentioned earlier in this book—is a three-part plan.

A lot of people try the "exercise-only" approach to losing body fat, believing that the more they work out, the safer they are when it comes to eating whatever they want and sacrificing as little as possible in their diets. That sort of wishful thinking isn't how a boxer prepares for a fight or a model prepares for a show, and it's definitcly not how you should prepare your body in order to become Sleekified.

Making the right changes to your diet is an essential part of the Sleekify program, since it accelerates how quickly you shed fat and show off that leaner, defined physique underneath—a body you've worked hard for and are proud of.

THE SLEEKIFY DIET—IT'S SIMPLER THAN YOU THINK

I'm the same weight today that I was twenty-five years ago, despite being twice as old and no longer fighting professionally. The reason: Beyond staying active, I still put as much thought into what I put in my body now as I did back then.

Every day, you have a variety of nutritional decisions in front of you—decisions that determine if you will fail or succeed with Sleekify. Make enough poor choices and you could easily undo what my program can help you achieve. However, make enough right choices and you'll quickly strip away even more fat, develop more lean muscle, and reset the rate at which you burn calories so you look even fitter and sleeker. After all, no one drops weight faster than a boxer in training.

Ask Yourself Why You're Eating

It's important to respect food, but many people do exactly the opposite.

I treat food as fuel. I know that when I wake up in the morning, I'll be teaching five to six sessions that day that will be physically demanding, so I make sure I give my body what it needs in order to survive and achieve for that day—and nothing more. And when I'm not teaching, my appetite adjusts accordingly.

If everything you eat, every bite you take, fulfills that purpose, then you're on the right track. But if any single bite you consume is for other reasons—such as out of boredom, to satisfy an emotional need, as a reward, or because you're accustomed to cleaning your plate instead of wasting food—then you're most likely consuming excess calories that your body doesn't really need.

If food is fuel, then what you end up doing is flooding your tank. There needs to be balance in your diet and a purpose behind each meal. That's why I recommend eating only between 1,200 calories (for women) and 1,500 calories (for men) daily while following the Sleekify program. Sticking with these guidelines, you'll be fueling up with only enough calories to match your energy needs for the program—and not a calorie more.

However, I realize that adhering to a diet of this size—especially since I'm not aware of how many calories you're currently eating—may be intense for some. If you feel that may be the case, then I need you to be aware of a few important things.

One, these guidelines are a target range that I'm hoping you'll hit,
there with you to make sure that you do. Ideally, for maximum results, this
to stick with, but the Sleekify high-intensity exercise program is so effective a
calories that even if you find yourself eating more calories than expected, you're
teed to see amazing results.

Two, once you've reached your fitness goals, know that you'll be able to reintroduce
more calories back into your diet on a regular basis, which I'll show you how to do in a
later chapter. If you keep in mind that the calorie change you're about to embark on is
temporary, it may help you find the strength to stick with it for the short term.

Make It "Natural"—or Say No to It

I've always been a "calories in–calories out" kind of person. But I also know that eating
a few hundred calories' worth of lean meat, fruits, and vegetables affects the body far
differently than eating a few hundred calories worth of candy, white bread, and soda.

Your body processes different foods in different ways, and the more unnatural, heav-
ily processed—or as I like to say, "man-u-fractured"—a food is, the more devoid it is of
nutrients, fiber, and other things that satiate your hunger, heal your body, and feed your
muscles. These types of foods may technically be fuel because they can provide energy,
but they're like fuel with sand mixed in. They simply sit in the body.

Instead, stick with clean foods that are packed with more nutrients for the body to
process. I have my clients try to eat food that's as natural as possible with either no preservatives or as few as possible. Basically: If it doesn't grow naturally from the ground
or above it, stay away from it. That means eliminating all processed, refined foods (such
as bagels, pretzels, processed rice, and pasta), refined sugar, sodas, fruit beverages,
cakes, cookies, and alcohol from your diet.

Mind you, this is what I would consider a dream scenario, and I understand that
being able to eat nothing but all-natural foods is a matter of convenience as well as af-
fordability. That said, if you don't have the option of eating all-natural foods all the time,
just know that this workout is so effective, it actually helps with your body's processing
and digesting of whatever food you do consume.

Time Your Meals Like Rounds

To maximize how efficiently your body processes your food, break up your daily caloric intake into smaller, more frequent portions throughout the day. This is a smart strategy for several reasons:

Larger meals raise your blood sugar levels, which can trigger an increase in the release of insulin within your bloodstream. Unfortunately, your body's response to all that extra insulin is to immediately store a greater portion of the calories you're eating as body fat.

When you eat five or six smaller meals and space them two to three hours apart, your body maintains a steady blood sugar level throughout the day, minimizing how much insulin your body releases so you don't store as many excess calories as fat.

It also provides your body with a steady stream of fuel that prevents you from bingeing—plus, your body burns a certain amount of calories just to digest food. By eating more often, you'll boost your metabolism more often just to process your food, so you'll burn off more fat and reveal more muscle.

Eat Your Largest Meal Three Hours Earlier

Most people eat the bulk of their daily calories in the evenings, around 5 to 7 P.M.—the exact time when they typically begin to relax and engage in less activity before eventually falling asleep. The problem is you're not really doing anything to burn off the calories you've just eaten when you consume them later in the day. In other words, you're fueling up your body when you've already reached the finish line—you're flooding your engine.

For me, I do a great deal of my work in the morning. So between 2 and 3 P.M.—around the time the average person may reach for a snack to satisfy themselves between lunch and dinner—I actually need more calories so I have enough energy to teach several classes between 6 and 9 P.M. Eating my largest meal between 2 and 4 P.M. works for my clients and me—and here's why.

In the morning, your metabolism is at its fastest, while in the evenings, your metabolism is at its slowest. Because of this, some people believe you should eat the bulk of your calories in the morning, then taper them off by eating less throughout the day

to stay in line with your metabolism. This can leave you feeling sluggish a
on, with less energy to devote to working out later (especially if the only tin
to exercise is in the evenings).

Eating on more of a bell curve—less in the morning, more in the midaft
then less at night—ensures that you'll always have energy to exercise without overt   .g
your tank with excess calories it has no choice but to store as fat while you sleep.

Think Before You Drink

Sipping water throughout the day—especially before, during, and after every meal—
can leave you feeling more satiated (so you're less hungry) and helps your body process
food faster as it absorbs even more nutrients from the foods you're eating. Being dehydrated can have the opposite effect, which can lower your work tolerance considerably,
causing you to put less effort into the Sleekify exercise program, or worse, possibly quit
from feeling too tired or weak.

Plain water is my main drink. I might have vegetable juice once in a while, and if I
have orange juice (which I'm prone to do because I tend to lean toward the sweet things),
I always cut it with seltzer water. But I take in only about a liter of water a day (roughly
33 ounces)—and that's being active. That's also about half of what's typically recom-
mended by nutritionists, who believe 64 ounces is the minimum one should drink each
day. But what I've noticed with people who want that "performance body" but can never
achieve it is that their bodies tend to hold on to water.

I know you might think: "Wait a minute! I can't even drink water?" But as a boxer,
when it's necessary to make weight in a month, or even with the women I train for the
Victoria's Secret show, it's important to cut back on water intake. It's a change that will
allow you to see more muscular definition under your skin.

If you're worried about not getting enough fluids, remember that your body draws a
large percentage of its water from the foods that you eat. The reason most people tend
to be dehydrated is that the majority of their diet is processed foods, many of which are
devoid of water. Because you'll be eating nothing but natural foods, such as fruits and
water-laden vegetables, your body will already be taking in an adequate amount of water
from your diet alone.

When you do drink, avoid any beverages with calories—including alcohol—and drink only water, plain tea (iced or hot), or plain coffee. That goes for diet and sugar-free drinks as well, since many contain artificial sweeteners and chemicals that can cause water retention. Finally, if water seems "tasteless" to you, try adding an all-natural flavoring, such as a squirt of lemon or lime juice or even a simple mint leaf.

Eat What You Want—When You Want It

Eggs are one of my favorite foods and a staple in my diet, but when I eat them is entirely up to my body. I never feel as if I have to eat specific foods at specific times throughout the day, such as having eggs for breakfast, a sandwich for lunch, and a salad for dinner. Instead, I let my body decide what it wants, when it wants it, so long as what it wants stays true to the amount of calories per day that I'm allowed to eat. That's why with Sleekify, I may offer guidance on how many calories and what types of foods you should eat, but when you decide to eat them is up to you.

That preconditioning to eat certain foods at certain times is something our parents (who may have meant well) and society have taught us, but I've never felt the need to eat as we've been programmed to do. So long as you're giving your body what it needs, keeping your calorie limit at the right level, and choosing all-natural foods, don't worry about what everyone else is eating. Instead, focus on what your body needs and wants each day.

Combine Your Foods for All-Day Energy

Whenever possible, try to have every meal be a combination of complex carbohydrates, protein, and healthy fats. To be more specific, each meal should be a mix of:

- A low-glycemic and/or complex carbohydrate (from fruits, veggies, and select grains, such as oats, brown rice, or quinoa)
- A high-quality protein (from low-fat meats, dairy products, or combining grains and legumes)
- Some form of healthy fats (from seeds, nuts, oils, or any type of fatty fish)

The reason: These three nutrients are broken down at different speeds by your body. By eating a mix in each meal, you'll give your body a sustained even flow of energy that will surprisingly leave you feeling fuller—oftentimes, you'll feel fuller than if you had consumed more calories of unhealthier foods that weren't a blend (which is how most people eat). This mix also makes you less likely to see a spike in your blood sugar levels, so your body will be less likely to store excess calories in your system as fat.

SLEEKIFY-APPROVED PROTEIN SOURCES

- Any type of lean meat or low-fat dairy product, including (but not limited to): chicken breast, cottage cheese, egg whites, any type of fish (Atlantic cod, flounder, grouper, haddock, halibut, sea bass, and trout, for example), pork (lean), protein powder, red meat (lean), skim milk, turkey breast, and yogurt.

SLEEKIFY-APPROVED CARBOHYDRATE SOURCES

- Any type of vegetable, including (but not limited to): asparagus, broccoli, Brussels sprouts, cabbage, carrots, cauliflower, celery, cucumber, edamame, eggplant, green beans, kale, lettuce, mushrooms, onions, peppers, spinach, squash, and tomatoes.
- Any type of whole fruit, including (but not limited to): apples, apricots, bananas, blackberries, blueberries, cantaloupe, cherries, dates, figs, grapes, grapefruits, green apples, guava, kiwis, mangos, melon, oranges, papayas, peaches, pears, pineapples, plums, pomegranates, raspberries, strawberries, tangerines, and watermelon.
- Any type of bean or whole grain, including (but not limited to): black beans, brown rice, cannellini beans, chickpeas, kidney beans, lentils, lima beans, pinto beans, quinoa, steel-cut oats, whole-wheat bread, and wild rice.

SLEEKIFY-APPROVED FAT SOURCES

- Any type of nut, seed, or fatty fish, including (but not limited to): almonds, avocados, Brazil nuts, cashews, flaxseed oil, hazelnuts, olive oil, olives, peanuts, pecans, pine nuts, pumpkin seeds, salmon, sunflower seeds, tuna, and walnuts.

Your Sleekify Seven-Day Meal Plan

Because I don't believe in eating by the rules—meaning, eating certain types of foods at certain times of the day—neither should you. However, I also realize that some people may feel more comfortable eating that way. That said, here are a few recommendations on just a few types of 250- to 350-calorie meals you can create using a mix of my Sleekify-approved foods:

SLEEKIFIED BREAKFAST OPTIONS

- 1 serving of Greek yogurt with a small handful of raspberries and $1/2$ whole-wheat bagel (300 calories)
- An egg-white omelet (made with 4 egg whites), one handful of spinach, $1/2$ tomato (chopped), one handful of chopped onion, and 1 oz. goat or feta cheese (250 calories)
- 1 protein shake (one scoop) using $1/2$ cup soy milk and $1/2$ banana (275 calories)
- $1/4$ cup steel-cut oatmeal with strawberries and 4 egg whites (250 calories)
- 1 protein shake (one scoop) using water and 1 tbsp. all-natural peanut butter (200 calories)
- An egg-white omelet (made with 3 egg whites) with $1/2$ cup chopped veggies, $1/2$ grapefruit, and 1 cup skim milk (225 calories)
- 4 oz. nonfat cottage cheese, $1/2$ cup pineapple chunks, and 10 to 12 almonds (225 calories)

SLEEKIFIED LUNCH OPTIONS

- 3 oz. chicken breast with a slice of low-fat Swiss cheese, 1 slice of avocado, and 1 slice of tomato—all wrapped in a large piece of dark-leaf lettuce (250 calories)
- 1 can of tuna (low-sodium and packed in water) mixed with 1 cucumber (diced) stuffed in a whole-wheat pita (300 calories)
- 4 oz. sliced beef tenderloin, 2 cups mixed greens, and 1 tsp. olive oil (275 calories)
- 1 protein smoothie—mix one semi-frozen bag of fruit, 8 oz. nonfat Greek yogurt, and a dozen almonds (275 calories)

- ¼ cup steel-cut oats mixed with ½ pear (sliced in chunks), ½ oz. chopped almonds, and ½ tbsp. raw honey (300 calories)
- ½ cup vegetarian chili topped with 1 oz. grated cheddar cheese (250 calories)
- Salmon and avocado sushi roll (300 calories)

SLEEKIFIED DINNER OPTIONS

- 4 oz. baked trout, ⅓ cup quinoa, and ½ cup green beans (275 calories)
- 4 oz. sirloin round steak on a bed of arugula, 1 chopped tomato, and 1 tbsp. sunflower seeds (300 calories)
- 3 oz. chicken breast (grilled), ½ cup brown rice, and 1 cup steamed broccoli (300 calories)
- 3 oz. thinly sliced rib steak, 1 oz. mozzarella cheese, and 1 tomato sliced, drizzled with 1 tsp. olive oil and 1 tsp. balsamic vinegar (250 calories)
- 4 oz. roasted pork tenderloin served with ⅓ cup long-grain rice and 4 oz. asparagus (275 calories)
- 3 oz. broiled tuna, one medium-sized sweet potato, and ⅓ cup snow peas (250 calories)
- ½ cup black beans mixed with ⅓ cup brown rice and ½ cup chopped vegetables—bell peppers, onions, and tomatoes (250 calories)

SLEEKIFIED SNACK OPTIONS

- 1 medium-sized apple, 8–10 raw walnuts, and 3 egg whites (275 calories)
- 1 cup sliced peppers, celery, and baby carrots, 2 egg whites, and 2 tbsp. hummus (200 calories)
- 4 large stalks of celery topped with 2 tbsp. all-natural peanut butter (250 calories)
- 1 cup edamame and a piece of whole-grain toast (275 calories)
- 1 stick of string cheese, 1 orange, and 1 tbsp. pumpkin seeds (200 calories)
- 1½ cups air-popped popcorn and 1 tbsp. cashews (225 calories)
- ¾ cup grapes, ½ cup almond milk, and 1 oz. peanuts (275 calories)

AERO-TIP—Stay within your comfort zone. Spinach may be healthy for you and a great water-laden, low-calorie vegetable, but it's helpful to your body only if it can make it past your mouth. Instead of forcing yourself to eat every type of healthier fare, don't be afraid to stick with the few foods you know you'll eat, even if that ends up being a limited few.

AERO-TIP—Know what 100 looks like. The next time you're eating, measure out exactly 100 calories of whatever natural food you're about to eat, then write down that size—or take a quick picture of it on your phone. Having a visual reference of what 100 calories physically looks like of the types of foods you'll be eating often can give you a rough idea of how much you're consuming during each meal.

AERO-TIP—Charge up before you sweat it out. If you're not caffeine-sensitive, try taking 100–150 milligrams of caffeine—the amount you get from a large cup of plain coffee—sixty minutes prior to your workout. The extra caffeine will help mobilize the free fatty acids in your blood, causing your body to use more fat as fuel instead of glycogen (the stored carbohydrates in your body that your body relies on for energy). The end result: You'll burn more fat, plus have more glycogen to use for longer, stronger workouts.

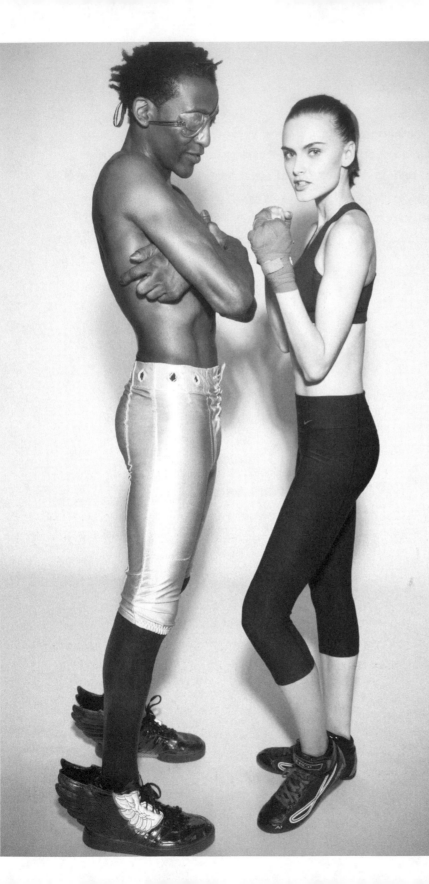

FOUR

SLEEKIFY: YOUR MIND—THE MENTAL EDGE

I N A FIGHT WITH YOUR BODY, YOU MUST EMPLOY YOUR MIND.

Sleekify isn't just a workout for your muscles—it's a workout for your mind, an aspect that's missing from many of the exercise books, programs, and fitness regimes you may have tried in the past.

There are plenty of people with amazing physical abilities in this world—those who are more powerful, faster, more agile, more resilient, and so forth than the majority. But we've all seen athletes win without a surplus of these attributes, just as often as we've watched incredible athletes we always thought were destined for greatness never fulfill the promise of their abilities.

The reason in many cases is simple: Whether you're an athlete, artist, musician, mathematician, politician, or anyone who's ever wanted to achieve something that's out of reach, the only hope you have to be able to achieve that goal is through one thing: sacrifice.

If you're not willing to sacrifice in order to achieve your goal, you're merely engaging your body, not your mind—which leaves you running at 50 percent capacity. Sacrifice allows you to clear your vision of distractions and focus on the task at hand. It's a departure from convenience and what's comfortable—it's a departure from what you know.

It means giving 100 percent of yourself to the cause with no regrets should you not achieve what you've set out to achieve.

But mostly, it's what gives you your best chance, maybe your only chance, to win in this fight to reclaim and Sleekify your body.

Fighters recognize the importance of honing their mental edge. When a fighter steps into the ring in the best shape of their life, they may be stronger, faster, and more agile than their opponent, but if they lack heart, if they lack drive, if they lack the ability to get knocked down and get back up—they can easily lose the fight.

Sometimes, all it takes is one unexpected blow, one punch to the gut that you never saw coming that causes you to quit instead of continuing to persevere. It doesn't matter that you still possess the tools to win. It doesn't matter if you're the greatest fighter in the world. Because there is no amount of money or fame that will win it for you—you have to want to win it for yourself.

I'M YOUR CORNERMAN NOW

Remember what I said at the beginning of this book: The reason boxers have "cornermen" (those coaches who circle a fighter between rounds to assist them during a fight) isn't just to get a drink of water and have their cuts mended.

It's to get strategic guidance and emotional support. Cornermen help their fighters put everything aside that may be distracting them, as well as correct them on what they're doing wrong, so they can focus on the next round. The fighter may be the captain of the ship, but the cornermen act as the navigational specialists who make traveling the treacherous ocean that much easier. It's that mentality, that knowledge of self and human instinct, that is essential to win a fight—and that includes winning a fight against yourself.

In boxing, your opponent may know all of your strengths and all of your weaknesses. When it comes to succeeding with Sleekify, you need to understand your opponent—and that's you. You need to have a defense for every offense—you need to be prepared mentally for every possible contingency you may throw at yourself.

That means looking at your own habits and what most likely may derail you from the program, then figuring out the best ways to block and counter them.

As your cornerman, I've got your back now—and these are some of the secrets I use with my clients to turn their hurtful habits into Sleekify-boosting behaviors.

Find Your Individual Incentive

Most of my celebrity clients have different reasons to stay slim. It could be getting a contract worth millions of dollars, being sleek enough to beat out the competition for a role or job, or excelling in their sport. For them, their very livelihood could be decided by what their bodies reflect.

If you're in a similar situation, then you've found your incentive. But if your paycheck isn't dictated by your physique, you may need something equally motivating to push you when you need that nudge. Tying the end goal—which will be a sleeker, fitter you—into another benefit that's just as (if not more) important than looking great can be the trigger.

I have clients who do it to stay youthful and active enough to play with their children. I have others who are driven because they want to improve their health and live a higher quality of life. I even work with clients who may be bored and do it purely for the challenge of proving to themselves that they can. There are so many reasons to get in shape beyond just the physical, but we each have at least one and that reason may be unique and yours alone. If you can find that incentive before starting Sleekify and tap into it, you'll be less likely to walk away before the program helps you reach your weight loss goals.

Accept Your Muscular IQ

No fighter is perfect. Every fighter has their strengths and every fighter has their weaknesses. Just as people have distinct IQs when it comes to their minds, they also have distinct IQs when it comes to their muscles.

Because I've never had the pleasure of meeting you, I don't know what your muscular IQ is (which I consider to be how you may be able to articulate your muscles, while working at various speeds and remembering select combinations). But I do know this: There are a rare few with a high muscular IQ who can pick up every exercise with ease and have no problem getting the hang of every movement, maneuver, and drill in Sleekify.

You may need more practice, not because you can't do what's been asked of you, or because you're not trying, but because your body isn't as quick to understand what's being asked of it. That's all. You may find it challenging to perform certain exercises at a certain speed or find yourself tripping over the rope more than you're jumping over it, but know that that is entirely normal.

As with anything in life, there's a certain amount of repetition that you have to invest in order to make something your own. Repetition is the mother of learning, but everybody learns differently and at their own pace. The more you practice Sleekify, the more coordinated and fit you'll become. But know in the meantime, that so long as you're always trying your absolute best, you'll always make the best gains—no matter how many times you may slip or stumble.

Recognize and Respect the Sacrifice

There is a sacrifice that you have to make when following Sleekify, and, yes, it's necessary to make yourself feel uncomfortable. You have to be prepared for the three-part commitment of exercise, diet, and maintaining your mental focus. In other words, you have to be all in.

But to me, Sleekify is in a lot of ways like the sign for infinity, which is a loop that comes back around into itself. Meaning, what you put into it will always come back to you. If you put a lot of effort and energy into the program, you will get that effort and energy back because it's very much a cycle.

Accept that you will be out of your comfort zone, embrace it, and remind yourself that every ounce of energy you put in will come back to you. Remind yourself that it was being *in* your comfort zone for too long that led to the body you're presently not as happy with.

Build an Entourage Within Yourself

I told you I was your cornerman, but ultimately, the strongest individuals are the ones who can stand on their own.

You can surround yourself with positive people, which I won't deny is always helpful. When we're working toward a goal (especially weight loss), each of us has his or her own perspective—and yours may not be revealing everything to you.

You may not see or feel the changes within yourself immediately because that's the way our minds work sometimes. That's why one of the beautiful things about having supportive people around you is that they can see the differences and acknowledge each one. But it can also give you a false sense of confidence. Ultimately, when the bell rings, you are in that fight all by yourself no matter who is behind you. It starts with the individual. You need to listen to that little voice inside and you have to stoke that fire within to convince yourself that you can do anything you set out to do—because you can.

Congratulate Every Victory

An avalanche never starts as an avalanche. Before it becomes an unstoppable force, it begins as one tiny ice crystal—a tiny ice crystal that combines with a few more tiny crystals to form a snowflake. And as each snowflake combines with another, it eventually becomes something far greater than itself.

Even though the results you'll reap from Sleekify will be extremely fast and incredibly satisfying, weight loss is still a process that begins by starting small. You need to respect that process, and one way to have that process work to your advantage is through recognizing every milestone you make in Sleekify, no matter how small or insignificant you may think each one is.

The first time you're able to throw a punch without looking at this book for instruction, that's a victory. Every time you're able to jump rope for a second longer than you did the last time, that's a victory. Every time you stay true to the program instead of shaving off seconds and making things easier for yourself, that's a victory—and I want you to congratulate yourself.

As small as each of these victories may seem, each one helps build momentum within you. And as you begin to stack up each one on top of the other, all of a sudden, you're able to reach heights you never expected to climb.

Look at Soreness as Success

Exercise—especially the type of high-intensity program you'll follow in Sleekify—translates into stress, because that's what exercise really is. It's stress we willingly place on our bodies in order to force them to adapt and become leaner, healthier, stronger, and Sleekified as a result.

Through my program, your body is going to experience a whole new type of soreness and fatigue and a different appreciation for your muscles. But that feeling that may seem uncomfortable for now is the adaptation process at work. You are virtually teaching your body how to speak a new language through the movements, maneuvers, and drills within Sleekify. That soreness shouldn't make you want to quit, because it means you're doing it right. It means you're executing Sleekify to the level that's going to make a difference.

Turn Everything—Positive or Negative—Into Energy

Some trainers feel the best way to maximize the results of their fitness plan is to minimize the amount of stress their clients experience throughout the day. They may say things like "Learn to forgive more," or that holding on to negative feelings might cause you excessive tension and anxiety that could sabotage your exercise and diet routine.

But how people cope with stress is such an individual thing. Instead, I try to look at everything, both positive and negative, as fuel. If someone is behind you and supports you, then is the world a more perfect world? Is it one that allows you to get things done much more easily? Absolutely!

If all you have going right now in your life is a lot of negativity, it may take more of an effort, but it's possible to turn those bad experiences into the fuel that pushes you forward. Unlike positive energy, which can be used immediately, negative energy is energy that needs more processing, but it can be just as effective in helping you reach your goals.

Successful fighters do it all the time, taking negative experiences, such as an injury or some obstacle that others say cannot be overcome or an emotional event happening in their lives, and using them to their advantage. All it takes is acknowledging the negativity in your life, and then saying to yourself, "This is the way it is. I understand that. But it's also energy that can either propel me forward or push me backward—the choice of which direction it moves me is entirely up to me."

Accept That You'll Get Knocked Down

I'm being metaphorical here. I'm not sending you into an actual boxing ring anytime soon.

But in life, as in boxing, everybody loses a round—that's reality. You may even lose a couple of rounds in a row, and that's okay. But when you get knocked down, you have to get back up and come back again.

As I mentioned, exercise is stress to your body and your body handles stress in many ways. There are going to be times—maybe more often than not—that you're going to look for an excuse *not* to Sleekify. And that's okay.

To win a fight, you don't have to score every point or win every round—you just have to rack up enough of them. With weight loss, each day is like a round, and what wins each round is staying true to the program. Will you fall off your diet once or twice? Or maybe not put as much effort into your workout on a certain day? Possibly, because that's inevitable—that's called being human. But it's really about getting back in there and striving to win the next round.

And if you win enough rounds, you'll always win the fight.

Acknowledge That the Fight Is Forever

Getting in shape and losing weight is an ongoing journey—one that if you're serious about staying fit will be an ongoing journey for life. It's not just about being bikini-ready when you're in your twenties—it's what allows you to be able to confidently rock that bikini in your thirties, forties, fifties, or whatever age you decide.

It's easy to become complacent once you've reached your goals. For a fighter, holding on to the title they've won can be even more challenging than the long, arduous journey it took to reach the title in the first place. That's because certain things that once encouraged you to stay on the path are no longer present in your life. There was a hunger. There was a necessity. But when that need has finally been fulfilled—then what?

Once you've Sleekified, there will no longer be that out-of-shape body in the mirror that wishes it was leaner and fitter. You'll no longer be out of breath trying to perform certain activities and reminded that you need to keep exercising. You won't find yourself envying anyone else's physique because they will be too busy envying yours. In fact, don't be surprised if you've now become someone else's inspiration.

But being in the best shape of your life now doesn't mean you've reached the end of the road. You have to view your success with Sleekify as an opportunity to turn onto a new path—one that lets you enjoy the physique that's been hiding underneath, waiting to come out.

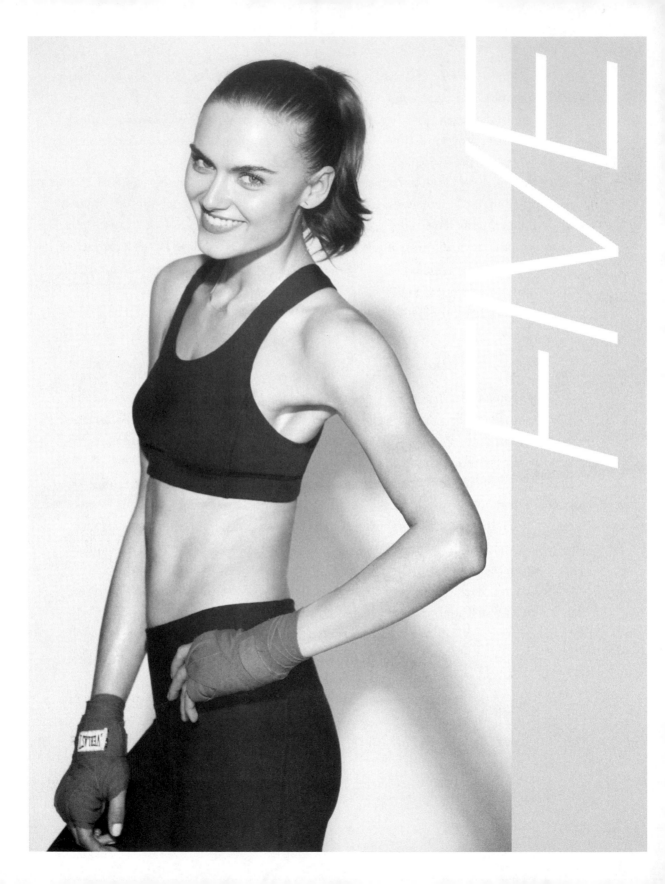

FIVE

WEEK ONE

WELCOME TO THE START OF THE SLEEKIFY TWENTY-EIGHT-DAY WORKOUT PLAN. Throughout the entire four-week program, you'll be exercising six days a week, performing a boxing-based routine that will range between forty-five and sixty minutes a session. You'll begin a new routine every three to four days (depending on where you are along the twenty-eight-day cycle), then switch to another routine after completing the workout for a straight three-day period.

With each routine, you'll follow it in the exact order as described. Trust me when I say that the order is important: It's designed in a way that lets you alternate between certain muscle groups—and between working your upper and lower body—to give portions of your body a much-needed breather.

Why the change-up every three days? I believe that you often get more out of an activity as you're learning it than after you've finally learned it. The human body and mind need to be in a constant state of being educated, which is easily done through changing things up and making things new again and more stimulating.

After three days, even though you may not have every move down, your body will still be adjusting to the routine. By completely changing things around every three days, Sleekify takes your body back to the start again, mixing things up to keep everything fresh for both your muscles and your mind.

BEFORE AND AFTER EACH ROUTINE

THE SLEEKIFY WARM-UP: Instead of immediately throwing punches and jumping rope, you have to do what I call a "stim" stretch (short for stimulation stretch) warm-up. The brief, nine-move, full-body warm-up you'll do before each session of Sleekify really isn't a stretching session as much as it is an awakening of your body.

Your muscles need to be reminded that they are about to participate in fast exercise. Picture a cat waking up from its nap. It stretches, then slowly begins to move, until eventually, it's able to react and move at high speeds. Being able to move your joints through their complete range of motion will improve your overall performance in Sleekify, as well as improve your coordination and balance.

The Sleekify Cooldown: After you finish the workout, you'll also be asked to do a short cooldown routine. As much as you might want to skip this part—either because you're tired from the routine or feel a cooldown is not important—don't!

Stretching after you Sleekify (when your muscles are warm and pliable) will help loosen your ligaments (which naturally tighten after exercise) and make you less susceptible to strains and cramps. Your muscles will recover faster when you're at rest, so you stay on target to meet all of your exercise goals. It also helps improve and achieve a fuller range of motion, which is something most people lose as they get older.

SLEEKIFY WEEK ONE MADE SIMPLE

For Week One, you'll be doing two separate workouts. Once you begin each workout, you'll continue to use it each day for a total of three straight days before moving on to the next workout. After the six-day cycle is over, you'll rest on the seventh day before moving on to Week Two.

Each workout routine is broken down into three "rounds," where you'll be doing a variety of Aerobox, Aerojump, and Aerosculpt exercises and drills. As you move from exercise to exercise within each round, you will rest for only as long as it takes you to get into position. However, between rounds, you have the choice of resting for 60 seconds before starting the next round or keeping the intensity high by immediately jumping into the next round without any rest.

WHY CAN'T I EXERCISE ON DAY SEVEN?

As I mentioned earlier in the book, I'm not aware of your muscular IQ. I'm also not aware of your overall fitness level, so asking you to take a break from the high-intensity program one day a week is a suggestion. The rest is as much for your mind as it is for your body. When you give yourself a day off, oftentimes you approach exercise with a new set of eyes— or in this case, absence makes the heart grow stronger.

However, if you are an intermediate or advanced exerciser—and after trying the program for six days, feel you can handle more—then you can exercise on Day Seven. You can either repeat the last day of the routine you've just finished or start the routine you'll be doing the following week a day earlier.

DAYS 1, 2, AND 3

New Aero-Moves

WARM-UP

- Standing Tilt
- Back Bend/Forward Bend
- Biceps-Forearm Stretch
- Shoulder-Triceps Stretch
- Squat Stretch

- Ankle Circles
- Standing Calf Raise
- Jog (or Jump) in Place
- Tri Jumping Jacks

AEROBOX

- Jab
- Power Punch

AEROJUMP

- Basic Jump
- Speed Jump
- Downhill Jump
- Slow Aerojump

AEROSCULPT

- Basic Squat
- Jump Squat
- Lunge Squat

COOLDOWN

- Standing Tilt
- Back Bend/Forward Bend
- Biceps-Forearm Stretch
- Shoulder-Triceps Stretch
- Sprinter's Calf Stretch
- Kneeling Quad Stretch
- Knee Hug
- Lying Hip-Glute Stretch
- Hip Flexor Stretch

THE PROGRAM (DAYS 1, 2, AND 3)

THE SLEEKIFY 3-MINUTE WARM-UP	
Upper Body	
EXERCISE/STRETCH	**LENGTH OF TIME/REPETITIONS**
Standing Tilt	Repeat 4 times to each side (hold each portion for 5 seconds)
Back Bend/Forward Bend	Repeat 4 times to each side (hold each portion for 5 seconds)
Biceps-Forearm Stretch	Perform once with each arm (hold each stretch for 5 seconds)
Shoulder-Triceps Stretch	Perform once with each arm (hold each stretch for 4–5 seconds)
Lower Body	
Squat Stretch	Perform the stretch once for 10 seconds
Ankle Circles	Perform the move once with each leg for 10 seconds
Standing Calf Raise	Perform the exercise for 30 seconds
Jog (or Jump) in Place	Do for 30 seconds
Tri Jumping Jacks	Perform the 3-part move once for a total of 30 seconds (do each variation for 10 seconds)

ROUND ONE

AEROBOX			
TYPE OF PUNCH	**POSITION**	**SPEED**	**NUMBER OF PUNCHES (OR LENGTH OF TIME)**
Left Jab	Pyramid	DS	32
Left Jab	Pyramid	ES	64
Left Jab	Pyramid	FS	128
Right Jab	Pyramid	DS	32
Right Jab	Pyramid	ES	64
Right Jab	Pyramid	FS	128
Power Left	Pyramid	DS	32
Power Left	Pyramid	ES	64
Power Left	Pyramid	FS	128

Power Right	Pyramid	DS	32
Power Right	Pyramid	ES	64
Power Right	Pyramid	FS	128
Left Jab/Power Right	Pyramid	DS	30 seconds
Left Jab/Power Right	Pyramid	ES	30 seconds
Left Jab/Power Right	Pyramid	FS	60 seconds
Right Jab/Power Left	Pyramid	DS	30 seconds
Right Jab/Power Left	Pyramid	ES	30 seconds
Right Jab/Power Left	Pyramid	FS	60 seconds

AEROJUMP			
EXERCISE	**LENGTH OF TIME**		
Basic Jump	180 seconds		
Speed Jump	30 seconds (then rest 15 seconds)		
Speed Jump	30 seconds		

AEROSCULPT			
EXERCISE	**LENGTH OF TIME**		
Basic Squat	60 seconds (approximately 30 full squats)		

ROUND TWO

AEROBOX			
TYPE OF PUNCH	**POSITION**	**SPEED**	**NUMBER OF PUNCHES**
Left Jab	Orthodox	DS	32
Left Jab	Orthodox	ES	64
Left Jab	Orthodox	FS	128
Right Jab	Southpaw	DS	32
Right Jab	Southpaw	ES	64
Right Jab	Southpaw	FS	128
Power Left	Southpaw	DS	32
Power Left	Southpaw	ES	64
Power Left	Southpaw	FS	128
Power Right	Orthodox	DS	32
Power Right	Orthodox	ES	64
Power Right	Orthodox	FS	128

AEROJUMP			
EXERCISE	**LENGTH OF TIME**		
Downhill Jump	180 seconds		
Speed Jump	30 seconds (then rest 15 seconds)		
Speed Jump	30 seconds		
AEROSCULPT			
EXERCISE	**LENGTH OF TIME**		
Jump Squat	60 seconds		

ROUND THREE

AEROBOX			
TYPE OF PUNCH	**POSITION**	**SPEED**	**NUMBER OF PUNCHES (OR LENGTH OF TIME)**
Left Jab/Power Right	Orthodox	DS	30 seconds
Left Jab/Power Right	Orthodox	ES	60 seconds
Left Jab/Power Right	Orthodox	FS	60 seconds
Right Jab/Power Left	Southpaw	DS	30 seconds
Right Jab/Power Left	Southpaw	ES	60 seconds
Right Jab/Power Left	Southpaw	FS	60 seconds
(7-move combo) Left Jab, Power Right, Power Left, Power Right, Power Left, Power Right, Power Left	Pyramid	ES	Repeat 8 times
(same as above)	Pyramid	FS	Repeat 16 times
(7-move combo) Right Jab, Power Left, Power Right, Power Left, Power Right, Power Left, Power Right	Pyramid	ES	Repeat 8 times
(same as above)	Pyramid	FS	Repeat 16 times
(7-move combo) Left Jab, Power Right, Power Left, Power Right, Power Left, Power Right, Power Left	Orthodox	ES	Repeat 8 times
(same as above)	Orthodox	FS	Repeat 16 times

(7-move combo) Right Jab, Power Left, Power Right, Power Left, Power Right, Power Left, Power Right	Southpaw	ES	Repeat 8 times
(same as above)	Southpaw	FS	Repeat 16 times
(7-move combo) Power Left, Power Right, Power Left, Power Right, Power Left, Power Right, Power Left	Southpaw	ES	Repeat 8 times
(same as above)	Southpaw	FS	Repeat 16 times
(7-move combo) Power Right, Power Left, Power Right, Power Left, Power Right, Power Left, Power Right	Orthodox	ES	Repeat 8 times
(same as above)	Orthodox	FS	Repeat 16 times

AEROJUMP			
EXERCISE	**LENGTH OF TIME**		
Basic Jump	60 seconds		
Speed Jump	30 seconds		
Slow Aerojump	30 seconds		
Repeat this 3-move cycle 3 times for a total of 6 minutes.			

AEROSCULPT			
EXERCISE	**LENGTH OF TIME**		
Lunge Squat (left foot forward)	60 seconds		
Lunge Squat (right foot forward)	60 seconds		

THE SLEEKIFY 5-MINUTE COOLDOWN			
Before you start, catch your breath by walking in place or side to side for 1 minute, or until your heart rate comes down.			
STRETCH	**LENGTH OF TIME/ REPETITIONS**		
Standing Tilt	Repeat twice to each side (hold each portion for 10 seconds)		
Back Bend/Forward Bend	Repeat 4 times back and forth (hold each portion for 10 seconds)		

Biceps-Forearm Stretch	Perform once with each arm (hold each stretch for 10 seconds)		
Shoulder-Triceps Stretch	Perform once with each arm (hold each stretch for 10 seconds)		
Sprinter's Calf Stretch	Perform the stretch 4 times with each leg for 10 seconds each time		
Kneeling Quad Stretch	Perform the stretch twice with each leg for 10 seconds		
Knee Hug	Perform the stretch once for 10 seconds		
Lying Hip-Glute Stretch	Perform the stretch twice with each leg for 10 seconds		
Hip Flexor Stretch	Perform the stretch once with each leg for 10 seconds		

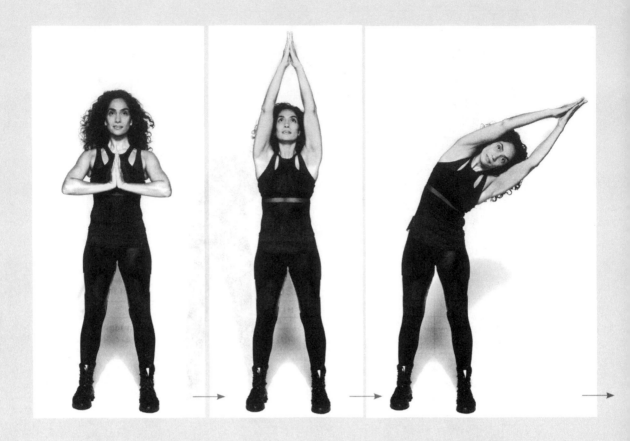

WARM-UP MOVES

STANDING TILT

Stand straight with your feet shoulder width apart and your palms pressed together in front of your chest—you should look like you're praying.

1.   Keeping your hands together, take a deep breath in and reach them up toward the ceiling as high as possible, keeping your arms straight as you go. You should feel this stretch under your arms and along the sides of your body.

2.   Slowly exhale and tilt your body to the left as far as is comfortable. You should

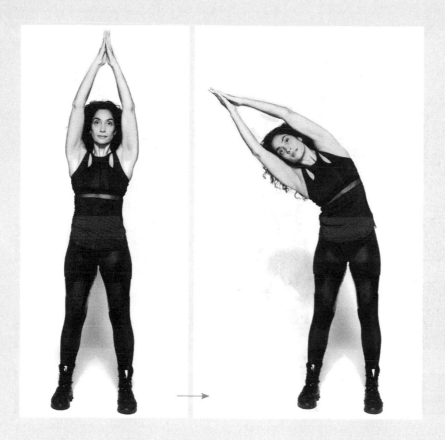

feel the stretch through to your obliques—the sides of your waist—at this point. Hold for 5 seconds.

3. Take a deep breath and come back to the original position. As you do, focus on reaching up as high and straight as you can.

4. Finally, slowly exhale and tilt your body to the right as far as it's comfortable. Hold for 10 seconds.

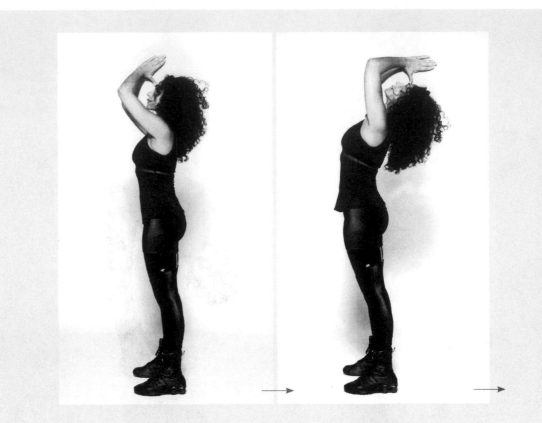

BACK BEND/FORWARD BEND

Stand straight with your feet slightly wider than shoulder width apart and place your thumbs on your forehead—your thumbs should be pointing downward with your elbows pointing slightly forward.

1.   Keeping your thumbs on your head, slowly tilt your head back as you curve your spine backward as far as is comfortable. (Don't challenge your balance—instead, bend only far enough where you feel you can hold the position.) Pause for 10 seconds.

2.   Slowly—and I mean *slowly*—return to a standing position as you reach your arms back behind you, lock your thumbs together, straighten your arms, and bend at

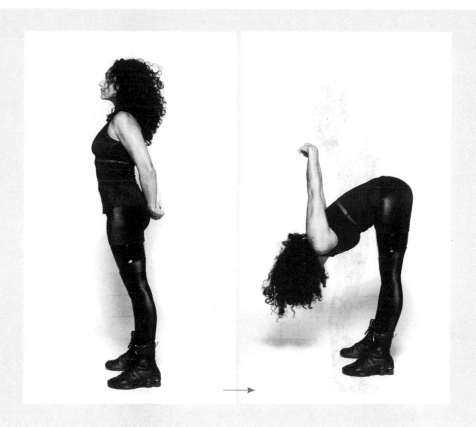

the waist all the way forward—your hands should end up pointing at the ceiling. Pause for 5 seconds.

3. Continue to alternate between leaning backward (thumbs on forehead) and bending forward (thumbs locked behind back) for the rest of the move.

NOTE: Remember to go into this move slowly. After the workout, you may be more prone to dizziness.

BICEPS-FOREARM STRETCH

Stand straight and reach your left arm out straight in front of you, palm facing the ceiling. With your right hand, grab the fingers of your left hand from underneath. Gently bend the fingers of your left hand down slowly until you feel a stretch in your fingers and forearms. Hold the stretch for a count of 5 and repeat with the opposite arm.

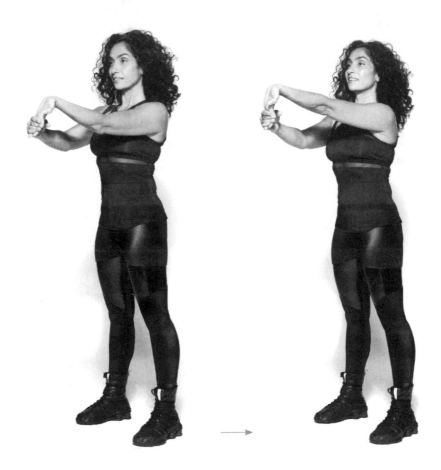

SHOULDER-TRICEPS STRETCH

Raise your right arm over your head, then bend your elbow so your right hand drops below your head. Place your left hand on top of your right elbow and gently pull your right arm toward your head. Hold the stretch for about 4 to 5 seconds, then repeat with the opposite arm.

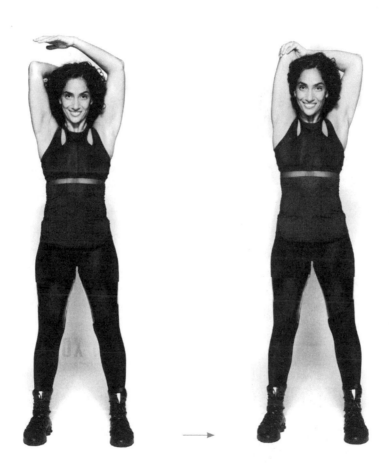

Stand straight with your arms down by your sides. Raising your heels, slowly sit back into a squat position, then rest one arm on top of your knees—placing your other hand between your knees and on the floor for support—and stretch for 5 to 6 seconds.

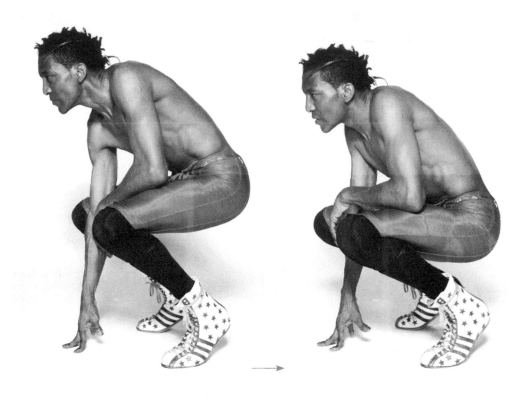

Get into a sprinter's stance: Place your hands on the floor about shoulder width apart. Extend your right leg straight behind you and place your right foot on the floor with your heel raised—only the ball and toes of your right foot should touch the floor. Your left leg should be bent, with your left knee in closer to your chest—again, your heel should be elevated so that only the ball and toes of your left foot touch the floor.

Holding this pose, gently press the toes of your left foot into the floor and begin circling your left leg—keeping your toes on the floor at all times—to help loosen up your left ankle. Rotate your leg for 10 seconds, then switch positions to repeat the exercise with your right ankle.

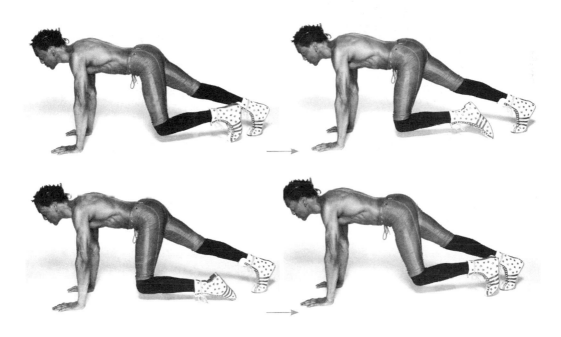

Stand straight with your feet hip width apart and either your arms down by your sides or your fists up by your chin. Rise up on your toes so that your heels come off the floor as far as possible. Lower yourself back down to the floor and repeat.

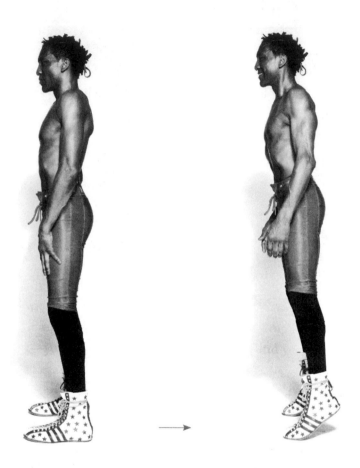

Stand in one spot and either lightly jog or jump in place at a light pace. Don't go all out—the purpose of the warm-up is to get blood into your muscles, not overtax them before they're ready to be challenged.

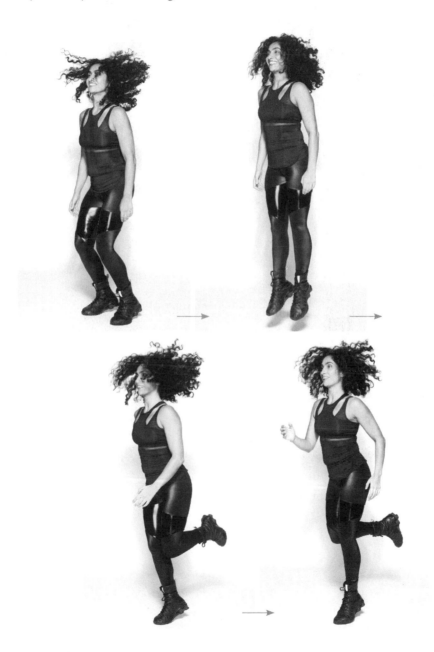

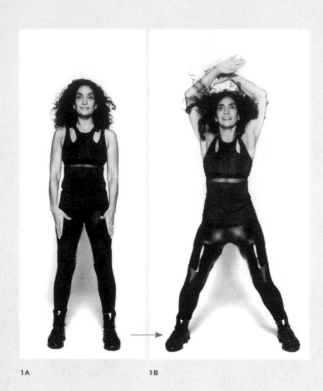
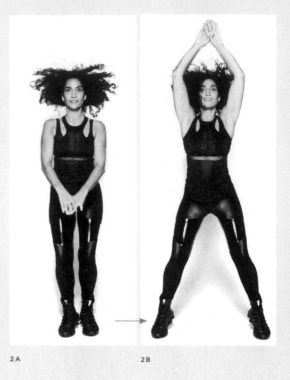

1A   1B   2A   2B

TRI JUMPING JACKS

For this warm-up, you'll do three types of jumping jacks—starting with a basic jumping jack—for 10 seconds each.

1.   Stand straight with your arms at your sides and your legs straight, knees unlocked. Quickly sweep your arms out from your sides and up above your head as you simultaneously jump high enough to spread your feet wider than shoulder width apart. Quickly reverse the motion by hopping back into the start position—this time, bringing your knees and feet together—and repeat.

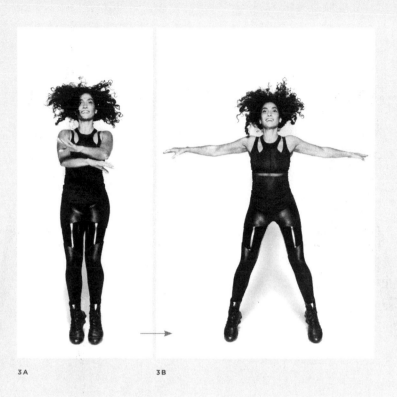

3A   3B

2.   With your legs and feet together, extend your arms out in front of your body and hook your thumbs. Quickly sweep your arms up above your head as you simultaneously jump and spread your feet. Quickly reverse the motion and repeat.

3.   Finally, with your legs and feet together, keep your arms extended straight out in front of you, but cross one arm over the other. Quickly sweep your arms out to the sides—keeping them at shoulder height—as you simultaneously jump and spread your feet. Quickly reverse the motion and repeat.

COOLDOWN MOVES

STANDING TILT

Stand straight with your feet shoulder width apart and your palms pressed together in front of your chest—you should look like you're praying.

1. Keeping your hands together, take a deep breath in and reach them up to the ceiling as high as possible, keeping your arms as straight as you can go. You should feel this stretch under your arms and along the sides of your body.

2. Exhale and tilt your body to the left as far as is comfortable. You should feel the stretch through to your obliques—the sides of your waist—at this point.

3. Take a deep breath and come back to the original position. As you do, focus on reaching up as high and straight as you can.

4. Finally, exhale and tilt your body to the right as far as is comfortable.

BACK BEND/FORWARD BEND

Stand straight with your feet slightly wider than shoulder width apart and place your thumbs on your forehead—your thumbs should be pointing downward with your elbows pointing slightly forward.

1. Keeping your fingers on your head, slowly tilt your head back as you curve your spine backward as far as is comfortable. (Don't challenge your balance—instead, bend only far enough where you feel you can hold the position.) Pause for 10 seconds.

2. Slowly—and I mean *slowly*—return to a standing position as you reach your arms back behind you, lock your thumbs together, straighten your arms, and bend at the waist all the way forward—your hands should end up pointing at the ceiling. Pause for 10 seconds.

3. Continue to alternate between leaning backward (thumbs on forehead) and bending forward (thumbs locked behind back) for the rest of the move.

NOTE: Remember to go into this move slowly. After the workout, you may be more prone to dizziness.

BICEPS-FOREARM STRETCH

Stand straight and reach your left arm out straight in front of you, palm facing the ceiling. With your right hand, grab the fingers of your left hand from underneath. Gently bend the fingers of your left hand down slowly until you feel a stretch in your fingers and forearms. Hold the stretch for a count of 5 and repeat with the opposite arm.

SHOULDER-TRICEPS STRETCH

Raise your right arm over your head, then bend your elbow so your right hand drops below your head. Place your left hand on top of your right elbow and gently pull your right arm toward your head. Hold the stretch for about 4 to 5 seconds, then repeat with the opposite arm.

SPRINTER'S CALF STRETCH

Get into a sprinter's stance: Place your hands on the floor about shoulder width apart. Extend your right leg straight behind you and place your right foot on the floor with your heel raised—only the ball and toes of your right foot should touch the floor. Hook your left foot along the back of your right calf—your left leg should be bent, with your left knee in closer to your chest.

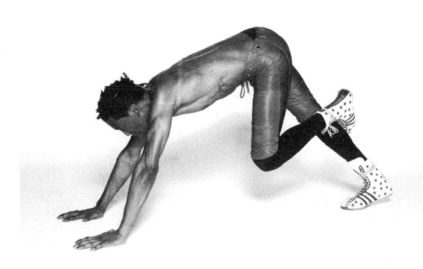

Holding this pose, gently push your right heel back until you feel a stretch in your calves. Hold the stretch for a few seconds and release. Then gently switch positions by extending your left leg back and hooking your right foot along the back of your left calf, and repeat the stretch.

KNEELING QUAD STRETCH

Get on all fours with your hands and knees touching the floor. Gently drop your left forearm to the floor for support, then reach back with your right hand and grab the top of your right foot. Gently pull your foot up and over your butt until you feel a stretch along the front of your right thigh. Your body should naturally tilt to the left—that's why it's key that your forearm remains flat on the floor to help balance yourself as you do the stretch. Hold for 8 seconds, then switch positions to stretch your left leg.

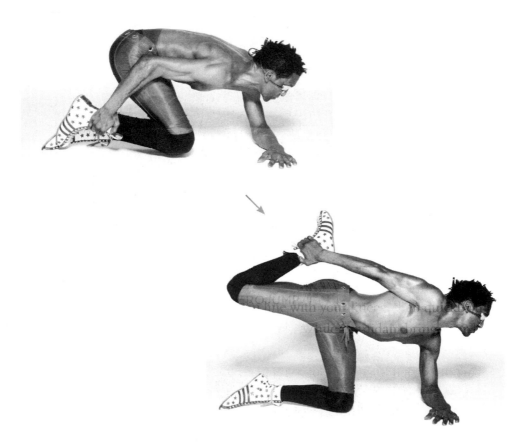

KNEE HUG

Sit on your butt with your legs bent and your feet flat on the floor. Wrap your hands around your legs, just below your knees. Slowly roll onto your back—keeping your arms wrapped over your knees. Gently pull your knees closer to your chest until your tailbone lifts off the floor. Hold the stretch for 10 seconds.

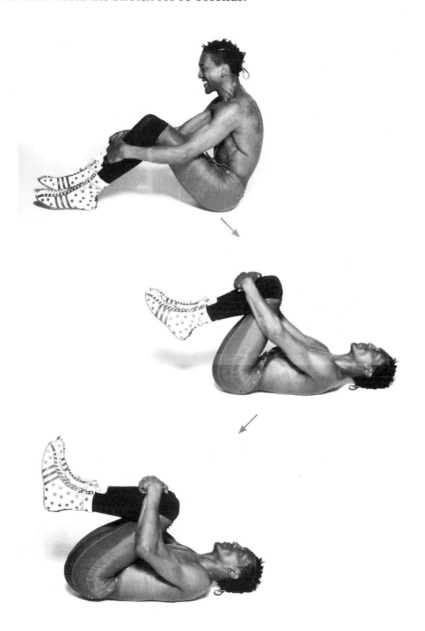

LYING HIP-GLUTE STRETCH

Lie on your back with your legs extended. Bend your right leg and bring your right knee up toward your chest, leaving your left leg flat on the floor. Wrap your arms gently around your right knee and hug it for 2 to 3 seconds (so that you feel a stretch along the back of your thighs and butt), then grab the outside of your right knee with your left hand and gently pull your knee across your body to the left as close as you can get it to the floor without lifting the opposite shoulder blade off the ground. Hold for 10 seconds, then release the stretch and repeat the move with the opposite leg.

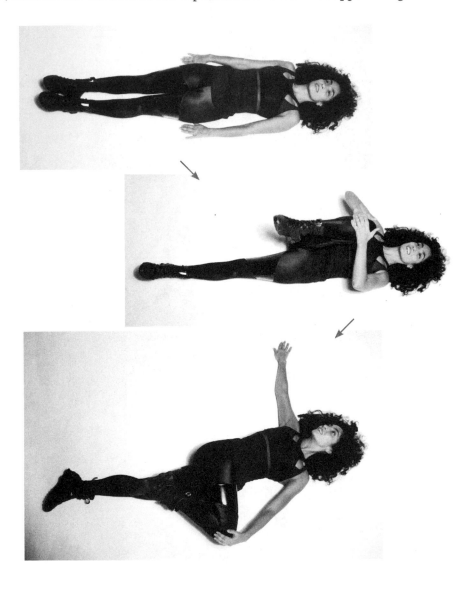

HIP FLEXOR STRETCH

Lie on your back with your left knee bent, left foot flat on the ground. Bend your right leg and rest your right ankle on top of the lower part of your left thigh. Take the palm of your right hand, place it flat along the inside of your right knee, then press your knee forward until you feel a slight stretch throughout your right hip flexor. Hold the move for 8 seconds, then switch positions to stretch the opposite leg.

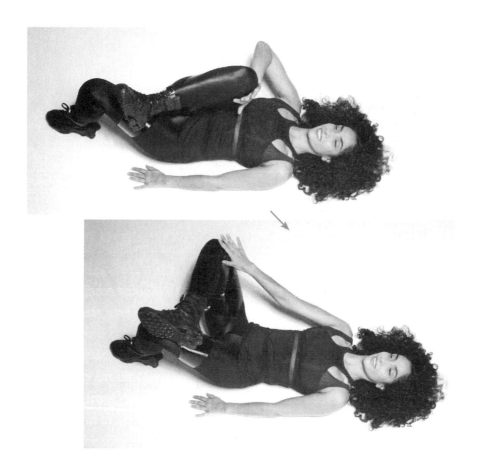

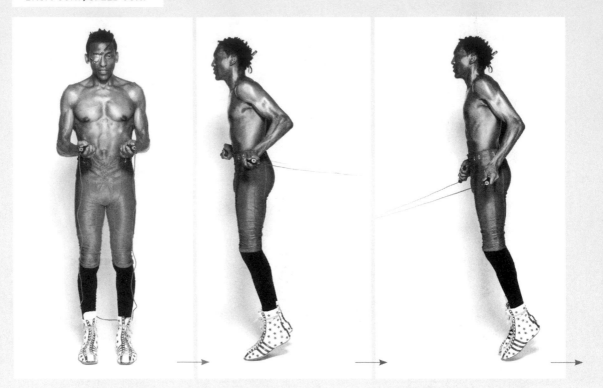

NEW AEROJUMP MOVES

BASIC JUMP

This beginner exercise works on your timing and coordination, which will help you master the other variations in the program.

START POSITION: Start by holding the rope at both ends—your arms should be down at your sides at waist level, palms facing the ceiling. Step forward so that the middle of the rope is right behind your heels.

THE MOVE: Keeping your hands close to your body, begin turning the rope forward, rotating only from your wrists. Once the rope comes down toward your feet, take a tiny hop—no more than an inch or so—to allow the rope to pass underneath you. Land on

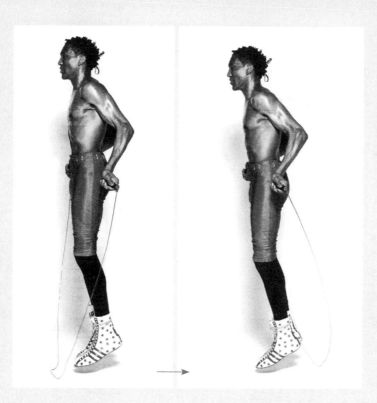

the balls of your feet—not flat-footed or on your heels (in fact, your heels should never touch the floor)—and repeat at a pace of roughly 138 rotations per minute.

SPEED JUMP

This variation adds a bonus to your calorie-burning efforts by also improving your hand speed, foot speed, and reflexes.

START POSITION: Start by holding the rope at both ends—your arms should be down at your sides, palms facing forward. Step forward so that the middle of the rope is right behind your heels.

THE MOVE: Keeping your hands close to your body, begin turning the rope forward, rotating only from your wrists. Once the rope comes down toward your feet, take a tiny hop—no more than an inch or so—to allow the rope to pass underneath you. Land on

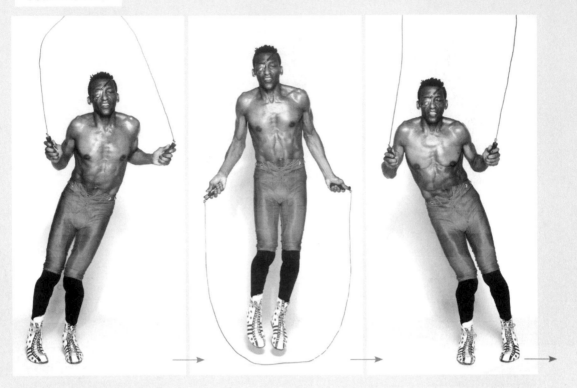

the balls of your feet—not flat-footed or on your heels—and repeat at a pace of roughly 150 to 156 rotations per minute.

Aero-Tips

- Although you're using the same technique as the basic jump, moving at a faster pace forces your body to become tighter to rotate the rope faster. You'll feel as if every single muscle in your body (your arms, your shoulders, your core muscles, and your legs) will become more rigid to allow you to hit that tempo.
- Don't be surprised that your jumps will be slightly lower to the floor. That's normal because to go faster, you must take smaller jumps so you don't waste as much time in the air.
- When doing a basic jump, you'll feel movement from your elbows through your fists. But at a speed pace, your elbows will lock to the body, so expect your hands and forearms to move a lot less.

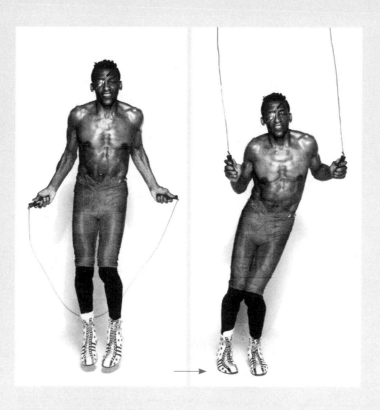

DOWNHILL JUMP

This variation has you hopping slightly from side to side, boosting your coordination while it simultaneously improves your overall agility.

START POSITION: Start by holding the rope at both ends—your arms should be down at your sides, palms facing forward. Step forward so that the middle of the rope is right behind your heels.

THE MOVE: Keeping your hands close to your body, begin turning the rope forward, rotating only from your wrists. Once the rope comes down toward your feet, take a tiny hop up and to the left (about an inch or two) as the rope passes underneath you. Land on the balls of your feet and repeat, only this time as the rope passes below you, take a small hop to the right. Continue jumping from left to right at a pace of roughly 138 rotations per minute for the duration of the exercise.

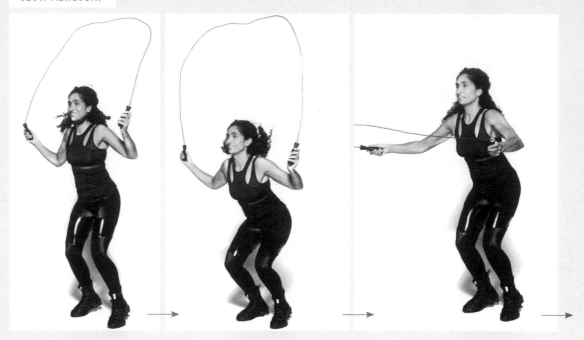

Aero-Tips

- Keep your legs and feet together and try to make each jump width-wise as small as possible. If you jump too far to the left or to the right, you'll find you won't be able to rotate the rope as many times per minute—plus, it increases the chances of the rope getting caught below your feet. As you become more comfortable with the move, you can start going a little bit wider than 1 to 2 inches.
- Your head should stay in one spot—not move with your body. You want your body to angle slightly to the left and right as you jump.

SLOW AEROJUMP

For this variation, you'll be moving at half the pace of the basic jump. Even though it may sound counterproductive to go slower than usual, bringing down the tempo keeps your quadriceps, glutes, and calves flexed for a longer period of time, which not only improves their muscular endurance, but also strengthens, shapes, and firms your legs from top to bottom.

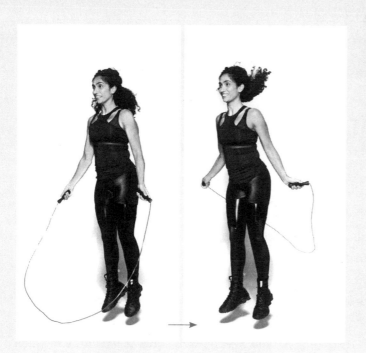

START POSITION: Start by holding the rope at both ends—your arms should be down at your sides, palms facing forward. Step forward so that the middle of the rope is right behind your heels.

THE MOVE: Keeping your hands close to your body, begin turning the rope forward, rotating only from your wrists. Once the rope comes down toward your feet, take a tiny hop—no more than an inch or so—to allow the rope to pass underneath you. Land on the balls of your feet—not flat-footed or on your heels—and sink down into a squat until your thighs are almost parallel to the floor. Push yourself back up and repeat at a pace of roughly 60 rotations per minute.

Aero-Tips

- Although you'll be staying on the floor twice as long as the basic jump, your legs should remain in perpetual motion and never stop the entire time. You shouldn't find yourself pausing at any point within the exercise.

- You may find yourself jumping up an inch or so higher than you normally do when doing the basic jump—that's fine, but don't leap any higher than that.

NEW AEROSCULPT MOVES

BASIC SQUAT

START POSITION: Stand straight with your feet shoulder width apart. Bend your arms and place your fists up along the sides of your face in front of your chin—your elbows should point down toward the floor.

THE MOVE: Keeping your fists locked in this position, quickly sit back and squat down until your butt is in line with your knees. Immediately push yourself back up into a standing position and repeat. It should take you 2 seconds to squat down and 2 seconds to stand back up.

Aero-Tip

- Focus on keeping the muscles throughout your legs (particularly your quadriceps, glutes, and calves) as well as your core muscles engaged (or flexed) the entire time. You'll see a shorter version of this tip in every single Aerosculpt exercise in this book for two important reasons: One, this helps protect your joints as you exercise, and two, it will guarantee that you'll thoroughly work your muscles each and every time, so you reach your goals even faster.

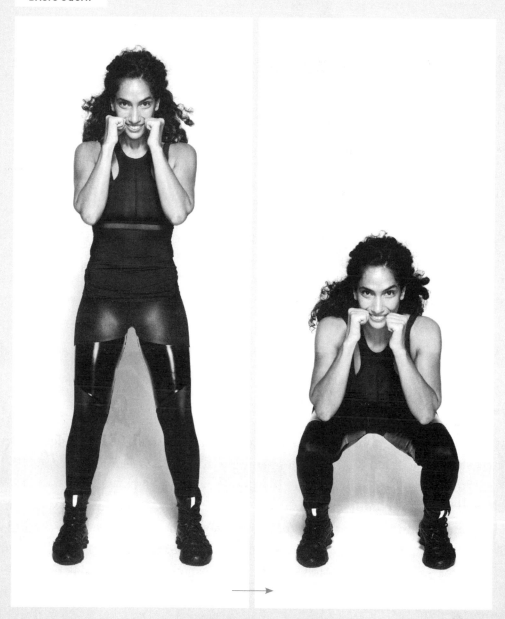

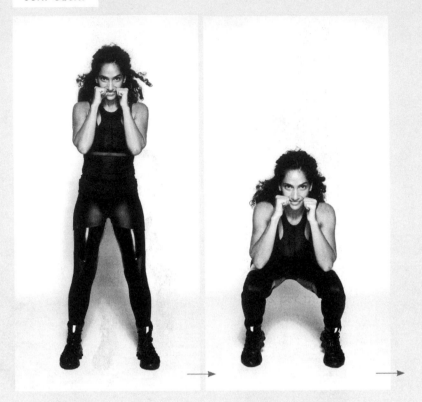

JUMP SQUAT

JUMP SQUAT

START POSITION: Begin in the same start position as the basic squat—feet shoulder width apart, fists by your chin.

THE MOVE: Squat down until your butt is in line with your knees, then quickly spring up into a standing position so that your feet come a few inches off the floor. Land on the balls of your feet, then immediately repeat the exercise. Shoot for a pace that has you performing a squat every 2 seconds—it should take about 1 second to sink down into the squat and 1 second to jump and land.

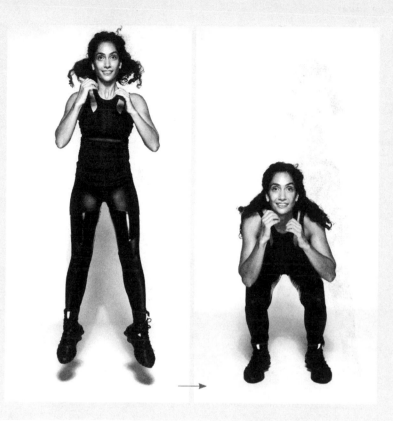

Aero-Tips

- Don't feel the need to jump as high as possible—it's not a contest to see how far you can hop off the floor. Instead, what you want to achieve more than anything is for your body to be moving in one continuous motion. That means the moment your feet touch the floor, you should immediately be sinking down into another squat—it should be a continual chain of movement from start to finish.
- Keep your quadriceps, glutes, calves, and core muscles flexed the entire time.

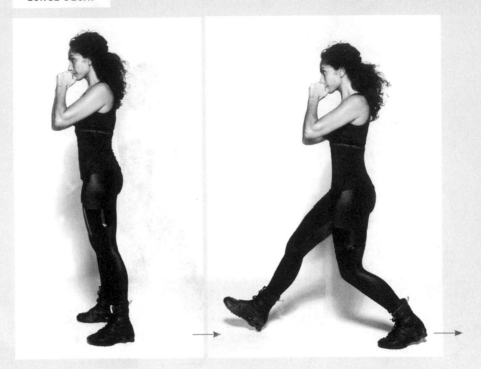

LUNGE SQUAT

START POSITION: Begin in the same start position as the basic squat—feet shoulder width apart, fists by your chin. Step forward with your right foot so that your feet are about 2 to 3 feet apart. Keep your right foot flat on the floor, but raise the heel of your left foot so that your weight is on the ball of your foot.

THE MOVE: Squat down until your right thigh is almost parallel to the floor—your left leg should be extended behind you with only the ball of your foot touching the floor. Push yourself back up into the start position and repeat, this time stepping forward with your

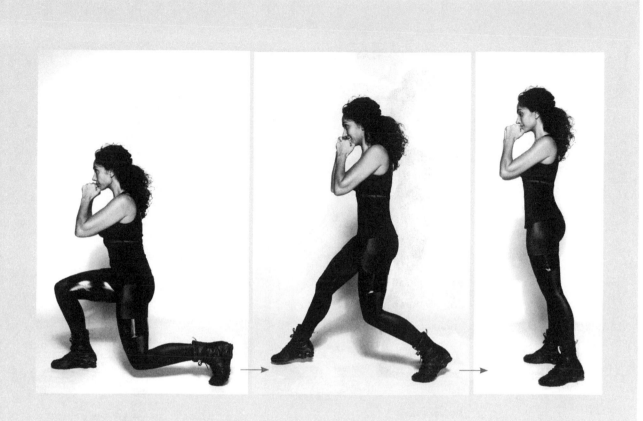

left foot. Continue to alternate between stepping forward with your right foot and your left foot throughout the exercise.

Aero-Tip

- Keep your quadriceps, glutes, calves, and core muscles flexed the entire time.

Past Aero-Moves to Expect

WARM-UP

- Standing Tilt
- Back Bend/Forward Bend
- Biceps-Forearm Stretch
- Shoulder-Triceps Stretch
- Squat Stretch
- Ankle Circles
- Standing Calf Raise
- Jog (or Jump) in Place
- Tri Jumping Jacks

AEROBOX

- Jab
- Power Punch

AEROJUMP

- Basic Jump
- Downhill Jump

AEROSCULPT

- (none)

COOLDOWN

- Standing Tilt
- Back Bend/Forward Bend
- Biceps-Forearm Stretch
- Shoulder-Triceps Stretch
- Sprinter's Calf Stretch
- Kneeling Quad Stretch
- Knee Hug

- Lying Hip-Glute Stretch
- Hip Flexor Stretch

New Aero-Moves You Need to Know

AEROBOX

- Double Jab
- Uppercut

AEROJUMP

- One-Leg Jump
- Aero Run
- Combinations

AEROSCULPT

- Downhill Squat
- Jump Change
- Slow Aero Ankle Touch

THE PROGRAM (DAYS 4, 5, AND 6)

THE SLEEKIFY 3-MINUTE WARM-UP	
Upper Body	
EXERCISE/STRETCH	LENGTH OF TIME/ REPETITIONS
Standing Tilt	Repeat 4 times to each side (hold each portion for 5 seconds)
Back Bend/Forward Bend	Repeat 4 times to each side (hold each portion for 5 seconds)
Biceps-Forearm Stretch	Perform once with each arm (hold each stretch for 5 seconds)
Shoulder-Triceps Stretch	Perform once with each arm (hold each stretch for 4–5 seconds)
Lower Body	
Squat Stretch	Perform the stretch once for 10 seconds
Ankle Circles	Perform the move once with each leg for 10 seconds
Standing Calf Raise	Perform the exercise for 30 seconds
Jog (or Jump) in Place	Do for 30 seconds
Tri Jumping Jacks	Perform the three-part move once for a total of 30 seconds (each variation for 10 seconds)

ROUND ONE

AEROBOX			
TYPE OF PUNCH	POSITION	SPEED	NUMBER OF PUNCHES (OR LENGTH OF TIME)
Double Jab (left hand)	Pyramid	ES	32
Double Jab (left hand)	Pyramid	FS	64
Double Jab (right hand)	Pyramid	ES	32
Double Jab (right hand)	Pyramid	FS	64
Double Jab (left hand)	Orthodox	ES	32
Double Jab (left hand)	Orthodox	FS	64
Double Jab (right hand)	Southpaw	ES	32
Double Jab (right hand)	Southpaw	FS	64
(7-move combo) Right Jab, Power Left, Left Jab, Power Right, Power Left, Power Right, Right Jab	Pyramid	ES	Repeat 8 times
(same as above)	Pyramid	FS	Repeat 16 times
(7-move combo) Left Jab, Power Right, Right Jab, Power Left, Power Right, Power Left, Left Jab	Pyramid	ES	Repeat 8 times
(same as above)	Pyramid	FS	Repeat 16 times
(7-move combo) Power Right, Power Left, Left Jab, Power Right, Power Left, Power Right, Power Right	Orthodox	ES	Repeat 8 times
(same as above)	Orthodox	FS	Repeat 16 times
(7-move combo) Left Jab, Power Right, Power Right, Power Left, Power Right, Power Left, Left Jab	Orthodox	ES	Repeat 8 times

(same as above)	Orthodox	FS	Repeat 16 times
(7-move combo) Right Jab, Power Left, Power Left, Power Right, Power Left, Power Right, Right Jab	Southpaw	ES	Repeat 8 times
(same as above)	Southpaw	FS	Repeat 16 times
(7-move combo) Power Left, Power Right, Right Jab, Power Left, Power Right, Power Left, Power Left	Southpaw	ES	Repeat 8 times
(same as above)	Southpaw	FS	Repeat 32 times

AEROJUMP			
EXERCISE	**LENGTH OF TIME**		
Basic Jump	60 seconds		
Downhill Jump	120 seconds		

AEROSCULPT			
EXERCISE	**LENGTH OF TIME**		
Downhill Squat	30 seconds		

AEROJUMP			
EXERCISE	**LENGTH OF TIME**		
Basic Jump	60 seconds		
Downhill Jump	120 seconds		

AEROSCULPT			
EXERCISE	**LENGTH OF TIME**		
Downhill Squat	30 seconds		

AEROJUMP			
EXERCISE	**LENGTH OF TIME**		
One-Leg Jump	180 seconds		

AEROSCULPT			
EXERCISE	**LENGTH OF TIME**		
Downhill Squat	30 seconds		

ROUND TWO

AEROBOX			
TYPE OF PUNCH	POSITION	SPEED	NUMBER OF PUNCHES (OR LENGTH OF TIME)
Left Uppercut	Pyramid	DS	32
Left Uppercut	Pyramid	ES	64
Left Uppercut	Pyramid	FS	128
Right Uppercut	Pyramid	DS	32
Right Uppercut	Pyramid	ES	64
Right Uppercut	Pyramid	FS	128
Left Uppercut	Orthodox	DS	32
Left Uppercut	Orthodox	ES	64
Left Uppercut	Orthodox	FS	128
Right Uppercut	Orthodox	DS	32
Right Uppercut	Orthodox	ES	64
Right Uppercut	Orthodox	FS	128
Left Uppercut	Southpaw	DS	32
Left Uppercut	Southpaw	ES	64
Left Uppercut	Southpaw	FS	128
Right Uppercut	Southpaw	DS	32
Right Uppercut	Southpaw	ES	64
Right Uppercut	Southpaw	FS	128
Left Jab/Power Right	Pyramid	DS	30 seconds
Left Jab/Power Right	Pyramid	ES	30 seconds
Left Jab/Power Right	Pyramid	FS	60 seconds
Right Jab/Power Left	Pyramid	DS	30 seconds
Right Jab/Power Left	Pyramid	ES	30 seconds
Right Jab/Power Left	Pyramid	FS	60 seconds
Left Jab/Left Uppercut	Pyramid	DS	30 seconds
Left Jab/Left Uppercut	Pyramid	ES	60 seconds
Left Jab/Left Uppercut	Pyramid	FS	60 seconds
Right Jab/Right Uppercut	Pyramid	DS	30 seconds
Right Jab/Right Uppercut	Pyramid	ES	60 seconds
Right Jab/Right Uppercut	Pyramid	FS	60 seconds

AEROJUMP			
EXERCISE	**LENGTH OF TIME**		
Aero Run	60 seconds (rest 15 seconds)		
Aero Run	60 seconds (rest 15 seconds)		
Aero Run	60 seconds (rest 15 seconds)		
AEROSCULPT			
EXERCISE	**LENGTH OF TIME**		
Jump Change	30 seconds		
AEROJUMP			
EXERCISE	**LENGTH OF TIME**		
Aero Run	60 seconds		
AEROSCULPT			
EXERCISE	**LENGTH OF TIME**		
Jump Change	30 seconds		
AEROJUMP			
EXERCISE	**LENGTH OF TIME**		
Aero Run	60 seconds		
AEROSCULPT			
EXERCISE	**LENGTH OF TIME**		
Jump Change	30 seconds		

ROUND THREE

AEROBOX			
TYPE OF PUNCH	**POSITION**	**SPEED**	**NUMBER OF COMBOS**
(8-move combo) Left Jab, Power Right, Left Uppercut, Power Right, Power Left, Right Uppercut, Power Left, Power Right	Pyramid	ES	Repeat cycle 8 times
(same as above)	Pyramid	FS	Repeat cycle 16 times
(8-move combo) Right Jab, Power Left, Right Uppercut, Power Left, Power Right, Left Uppercut, Power Right, Power Left	Pyramid	ES	Repeat cycle 8 times

(same as above)	Pyramid	FS	Repeat cycle 16 times
(8-move combo) Left Jab, Power Right, Left Uppercut, Power Right, Power Left, Right Uppercut, Power Left, Power Right	Orthodox	ES	Repeat cycle 8 times
(same as above)	Orthodox	FS	Repeat cycle 16 times
(8-move combo) Right Jab, Power Left, Right Uppercut, Power Left, Power Right, Left Uppercut, Power Right, Power Left	Southpaw	ES	Repeat cycle 8 times
(same as above)	Southpaw	FS	Repeat cycle 16 times

AEROJUMP

EXERCISE	LENGTH OF TIME		
Aero Run	60 seconds (rest 15 seconds)		
Aero Run	60 seconds (rest 15 seconds)		
Aero Run	60 seconds (rest 15 seconds)		

AEROSCULPT

EXERCISE	LENGTH OF TIME		
Slow Aero Ankle Touch	30 seconds		

AEROJUMP

EXERCISE	LENGTH OF TIME		
Aero Run	60 seconds		

AEROSCULPT

EXERCISE	LENGTH OF TIME		
Slow Aero Ankle Touch	30 seconds		

AEROJUMP

EXERCISE	LENGTH OF TIME		
Aero Run	60 seconds		

AEROSCULPT

EXERCISE	LENGTH OF TIME		
Slow Aero Ankle Touch	30 seconds		

THE SLEEKIFY 5-MINUTE COOLDOWN			
Before you start, catch your breath by walking in place or side to side for 1 minute, or until your heart rate comes down.			
STRETCH	**LENGTH OF TIME/ REPETITIONS**		
Standing Tilt	Repeat twice to each side (hold each portion for 10 seconds)		
Back Bend/Forward Bend	Repeat 4 times back and forth (hold each portion for 10 seconds)		
Biceps-Forearm Stretch	Perform once with each arm (hold each stretch for 10 seconds)		
Shoulder-Triceps Stretch	Perform once with each arm (hold each stretch for 10 seconds)		
Sprinter's Calf Stretch	Perform the stretch 4 times with each leg for 10 seconds each time		
Kneeling Quad Stretch	Perform the stretch twice with each leg for 10 seconds		
Knee Hug	Perform the stretch once for 10 seconds		
Lying Hip-Glute Stretch	Perform the stretch twice with each leg for 10 seconds		
Hip Flexor Stretch	Perform the stretch once with each leg for 10 seconds		

NEW AEROBOX MOVES

COMBINATIONS

Two or more punches in succession is considered a combination. When you are throwing punches in combination, I want you to pick a point of impact in front of your body. I like to visualize an image about nose height—that's where I aim every punch.

Every combination should be a series of punches thrown in succession and without hesitation. As you go, remember to pull your hands back as fast as they go out. Each combination is like sprinting with your arms and doing calculus with your mind—at the same time. You have to think and react fast, but the benefits are huge.

NEW AEROJUMP MOVES

Just as the name implies, you'll use only one leg instead of both to hop over the rope—a tweak that will drastically improve your balance, build explosiveness, and take your leg muscles to a higher level of fitness.

START POSITION: Start by holding the rope at both ends—your arms should be down at your sides, palms facing forward. Step forward so that the middle of the rope is right behind your heels.

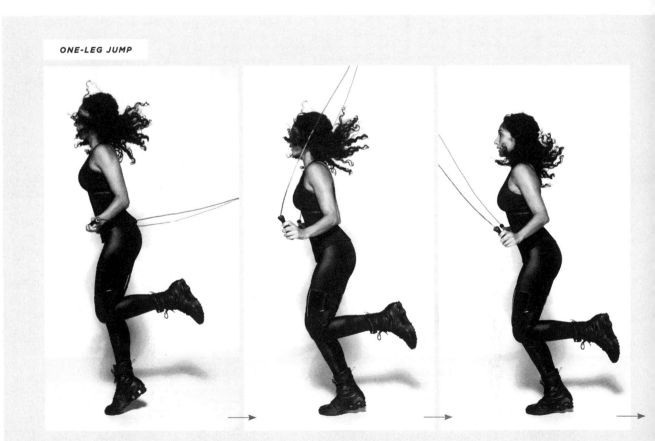

ONE-LEG JUMP

THE MOVE:

1. Keeping your hands close to your body, begin turning the rope forward, rotating only from your wrists. Once the rope comes down toward your feet, take a tiny hop with *both feet to start* to allow the rope to pass underneath you. Land on the balls of your feet and repeat for 8 jumps.

2. After the rope passes and your feet are in midair, raise your right foot behind you so you land on your left foot only. Repeat the exercise jumping over the rope using only your left foot—your right foot should stay raised behind you with your leg bent at about 90 degrees—for another 8 jumps.

3. While in midair, place your right foot back on the floor so that you're jumping with both feet again and repeat for 8 jumps.

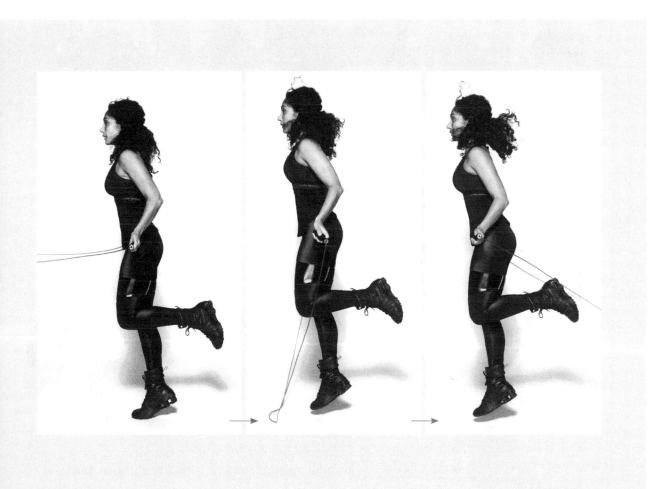

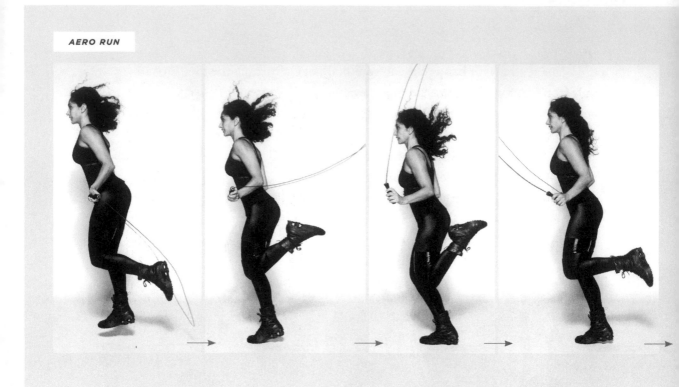

4.   After the rope passes and your feet are in midair, raise your left foot behind you so you land on your right foot only. Repeat the exercise jumping over the rope using only your right foot—your left foot should stay raised behind you with your leg bent at about 90 degrees—for another 8 jumps.

Aero-Tip

- For this variation, it's important that you perform it as dynamically as the basic jump—a pace of roughly 138 rotations per minute.

AERO RUN

This variation is basically an evolution of the one-leg jump, so you'll get most of the same benefits with a little bonus: more coordination and endurance.

You'll start by alternating between jumping on your left foot only for 8 jumps and your right foot only for 8 jumps. Once you have the timing down, you'll reduce the

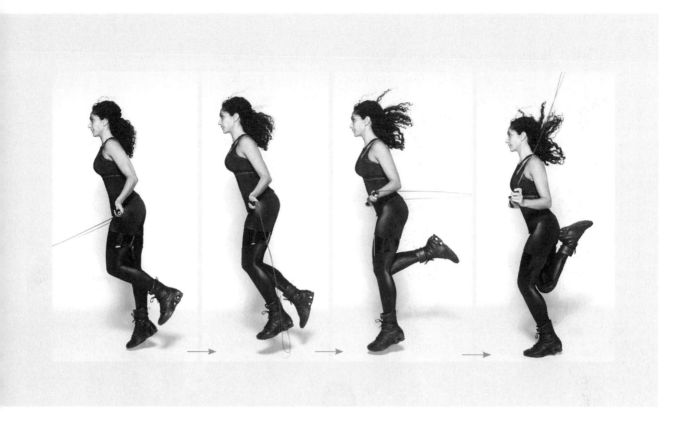

number of jumps per leg until you're eventually alternating from one leg to the other every jump.

START POSITION: Start by holding the rope at both ends—your arms should be down at your sides, palms facing forward. Step forward so that the middle of the rope is right behind your heels. Bend your right leg about 90 degrees so that your right foot is behind you and you're balancing on your left foot only.

THE MOVE:

1.   Keeping your hands close to your body, begin turning the rope forward, rotating only from your wrists. Once the rope comes down toward your left foot, take a tiny hop to allow the rope to pass underneath you. Land on the ball of your foot and repeat for 8 jumps.

2.   After the rope passes and your feet are in midair, switch feet by raising your left foot behind you so you land on your right foot only. Repeat the exercise using only your right foot—your left foot raised behind you—for another 8 jumps.

3. Repeat steps 1 and 2, only this time, do 4 jumps per leg.

4. Repeat steps 1 and 2, only this time, do 2 jumps per leg.

5. Repeat steps 1 and 2, only this time, do 1 jump per leg.

6. Continue alternating between jumping with your left foot only (right foot raised behind you) and your right foot only (left foot raised behind you) for the remainder of the exercise.

Aero-Tip

- Although the word *run* may make you want to sprint, stick with a pace of roughly 138–140 rotations per minute.

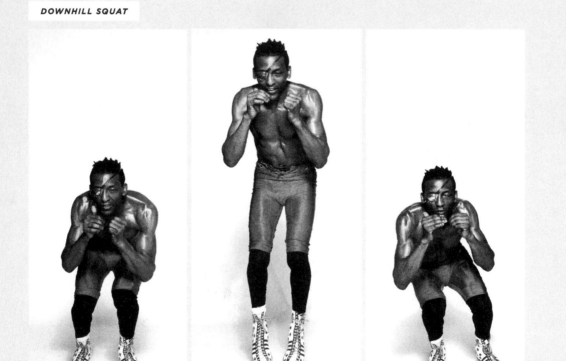

DOWNHILL SQUAT

DOWNHILL SQUAT

START POSITION: Stand straight with your legs together, knees and ankles touching—your fists should go up by the sides of your face just as if you were performing a basic squat.

THE MOVE: Keeping your legs together, squat down until your butt is in line with your knees, then quickly spring up off the floor just a few inches and laterally hop to your left. Land on the balls of your feet, then immediately repeat the exercise, this time hopping to your right. Continue to alternate from left to right throughout the exercise.

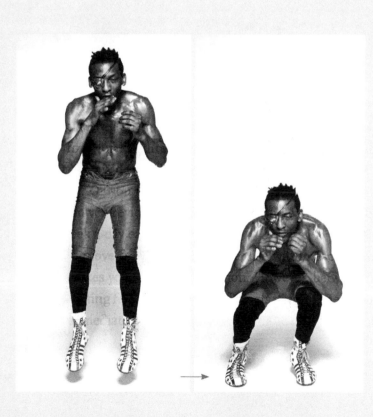

Aero-Tips

- Don't jump too high—the higher you go, the slower your pace will be and I need you performing the exercise as quickly as possible.
- Keep your quadriceps, glutes, calves, and core muscles flexed the entire time. Not only does it enhance the effect of the exercise; it also protects your ankles, knees, hips, and lower back.

JUMP CHANGE

START POSITION: Begin in the same start position as the basic squat—feet shoulder width apart, fists up by the sides of your face.

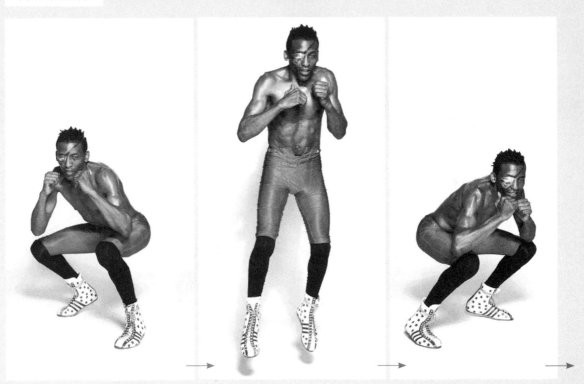

JUMP CHANGE

THE MOVE: Squat down until your butt is in line with your knees, then quickly jump up so that your feet come a few inches off the floor. As you come off the floor, simultaneously twist your entire body in midair to the left a full 90 degrees. (If you can picture standing in the middle of a clock—your feet pointing to twelve o'clock at the start of the exercise—your feet would now be pointing toward nine o'clock.)

Land on the balls of your feet, then immediately repeat the exercise, this time leaping up and twisting to the right a full 180 degrees so that your feet now face three o'clock. Continue to squat, jump, and twist from left to right throughout the exercise.

Aero-Tip

- Keep your quadriceps, glutes, calves, and core muscles flexed the entire time.

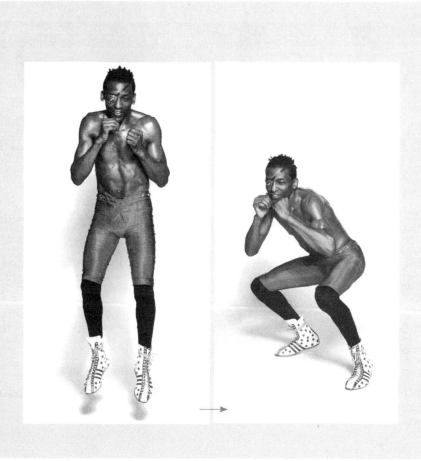

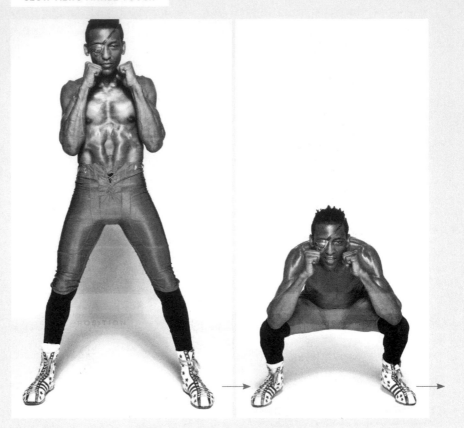

SLOW AERO ANKLE TOUCH

SLOW AERO ANKLE TOUCH

START POSITION: Stand straight with your feet slightly wider than shoulder width apart, fists up by the sides of your face.

THE MOVE: Squat down until your butt is in line with your knees, then quickly jump up so that your feet come a few inches off the floor. While in midair, bring your legs and ankles together so they touch, then quickly spread your legs back out—as you land on the balls of your feet, your feet should be slightly wider than shoulder width apart once more.

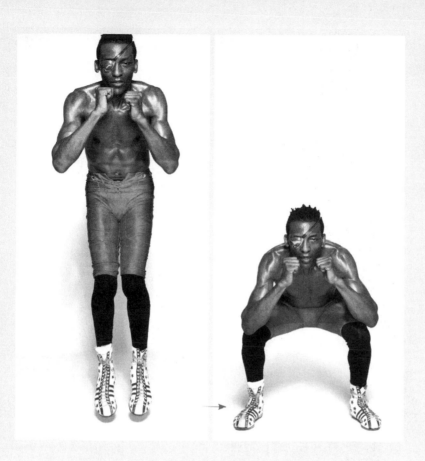

Continue to squat, jump, and touch/spread your legs before landing so that it remains one continuous motion throughout the entire exercise.

Aero-Tips

- Land on the balls of your feet at all times—your quadriceps and your calves are your shock absorbers, but in order for them to do their job right, you must allow your knees to bend every time you land.
- Keep your quadriceps, glutes, calves, and core muscles flexed the entire time.

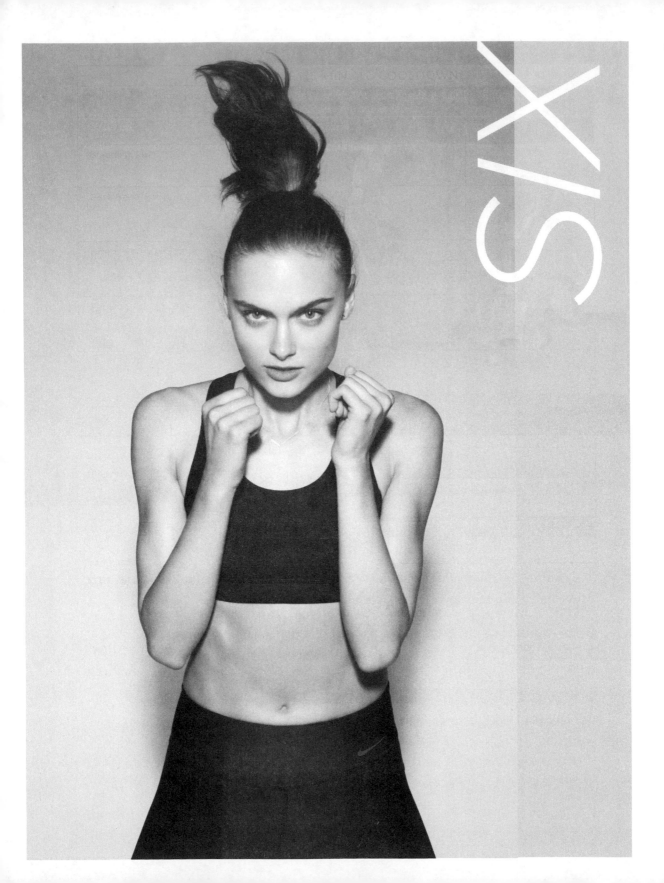

WEEK TWO

SLEEKIFY WEEK TWO MADE SIMPLE

FOR WEEK TWO, YOU'LL BE DOING TWO SEPARATE WORKOUTS, JUST AS YOU DID in Week One. Again, once you begin each workout, continue using it each day for a total of three straight days before moving on to the next workout.

After the six-day cycle is over, you'll rest on the seventh day before moving on to Week Three. Or you can add a seventh workout by either repeating the last day of the routine you've previously finished or starting whichever routine you'll be doing the following week a day earlier.

As you move from exercise to exercise within each round, you will rest for only as long as it takes you to get into position. However, between rounds, you have the choice of either resting for sixty seconds before starting the next round or keeping the intensity high by immediately jumping into the next round without any rest.

Past Aero-Moves to Expect

AEROBOX

- Jab
- Power Punch
- Double Jab

AEROJUMP

- (none)

AEROSCULPT

- Slow Aero Jack

New Aero-Moves You Need to Know

AEROBOX

- Hook

AEROJUMP

- Side-Under
- Side-Under (FAST)

AEROSCULPT

- Slow Aero Shuffle

THE PROGRAM (DAYS 8, 9, AND 10)

THE SLEEKIFY 3-MINUTE WARM-UP	
Upper Body	
EXERCISE/STRETCH	**LENGTH OF TIME/REPETITIONS**
Standing Tilt	Repeat 4 times to each side (hold each portion for 5 seconds)
Back Bend/Forward Bend	Repeat 4 times to each side (hold each portion for 5 seconds)
Biceps-Forearm Stretch	Perform once with each arm (hold each stretch for 5 seconds)
Shoulder-Triceps Stretch	Perform once with each arm (hold each stretch for 4–5 seconds)
Lower Body	
Squat Stretch	Perform the stretch once for 10 seconds
Ankle Circles	Perform the move once with each leg for 10 seconds
Standing Calf Raise	Perform the exercise for 30 seconds
Jog (or Jump) in Place	Do for 30 seconds
Tri Jumping Jacks	Perform the 3-part move once for a total of 30 seconds (each variation for 10 seconds)

ROUND ONE

AEROBOX			
TYPE OF PUNCH	**POSITION**	**SPEED**	**NUMBER OF PUNCHES (OR LENGTH OF TIME)**
Jab/Double Jab (left hand)	Pyramid	ES	30 seconds
Jab/Double Jab (left hand)	Pyramid	FS	60 seconds
Jab/Double Jab (right hand)	Pyramid	ES	30 seconds
Jab/Double Jab (right hand)	Pyramid	FS	60 seconds
Jab/Double Jab (left hand)	Orthodox	ES	30 seconds
Jab/Double Jab (left hand)	Orthodox	FS	60 seconds
Jab/Double Jab (right hand)	Southpaw	ES	30 seconds

Jab/Double Jab (right hand)	Southpaw	FS	60 seconds
Left Hook	Pyramid	DS	16
Left Hook	Pyramid	ES	32
Left Hook	Pyramid	FS	64
Right Hook	Pyramid	DS	16
Right Hook	Pyramid	ES	32
Right Hook	Pyramid	FS	64

AEROJUMP			
EXERCISE	LENGTH OF TIME		
Side-Under	180 seconds		

AEROSCULPT			
EXERCISE	LENGTH OF TIME		
Slow Aero Jack	30 seconds		

AEROJUMP			
EXERCISE	LENGTH OF TIME		
Side-Under	180 seconds		

AEROSCULPT			
EXERCISE	LENGTH OF TIME		
Slow Aero Jack	30 seconds		

AEROJUMP			
EXERCISE	LENGTH OF TIME		
Side-Under	180 seconds		

AEROSCULPT			
EXERCISE	LENGTH OF TIME		
Slow Aero Jack	30 seconds		

ROUND TWO

AEROBOX			
TYPE OF PUNCH	POSITION	SPEED	NUMBER OF PUNCHES (OR LENGTH OF TIME)
(4-move combo) ALL LEFT HAND: Jab, uppercut, hook, jab	Pyramid	DS	Repeat cycle 4 times
(same as above)	Pyramid	ES	Repeat cycle 8 times
(same as above)	Pyramid	FS	Repeat cycle 32 times

(same as above)	Orthodox	DS	Repeat cycle 4 times
(same as above)	Orthodox	ES	Repeat cycle 8 times
(same as above)	Orthodox	FS	Repeat cycle 32 times
(4-move combo) ALL RIGHT HAND: Jab, uppercut, hook, jab	Pyramid	DS	Repeat cycle 4 times
(same as above)	Pyramid	ES	Repeat cycle 8 times
(same as above)	Pyramid	FS	Repeat cycle 32 times
(same as above)	Southpaw	DS	Repeat cycle 4 times
(same as above)	Southpaw	ES	Repeat cycle 8 times
(same as above)	Southpaw	FS	Repeat cycle 32 times

AEROJUMP			
EXERCISE	LENGTH OF TIME		
Side-Under	180 seconds		

AEROSCULPT			
EXERCISE	LENGTH OF TIME		
Slow Aero Shuffle	30 seconds		

AEROJUMP			
EXERCISE	LENGTH OF TIME		
Side-Under	180 seconds		

AEROSCULPT			
EXERCISE	LENGTH OF TIME		
Slow Aero Shuffle	30 seconds		

AEROJUMP			
EXERCISE	LENGTH OF TIME		
Side-Under (FAST)	180 seconds		

AEROSCULPT			
EXERCISE	LENGTH OF TIME		
Slow Aero Shuffle	30 seconds		

ROUND THREE

AEROBOX			
TYPE OF PUNCH	**POSITION**	**SPEED**	**NUMBER OF PUNCHES (OR LENGTH OF TIME)**
(8-move combo) Power Left, Power Right, Left Uppercut, Right Uppercut, Left Hook, Right Hook, Power Left, Power Right	Pyramid	ES	Repeat cycle 8 times
(same as above)	Pyramid	FS	Repeat cycle 32 times
(same as above)	Orthodox	ES	Repeat cycle 8 times
(same as above)	Orthodox	FS	Repeat cycle 32 times
(8-move combo) Power Right, Power Left, Right Uppercut, Left Uppercut, Right Hook, Left Hook, Power Right, Power Left	Pyramid	ES	Repeat cycle 8 times
(same as above)	Pyramid	ES	Repeat cycle 8 times
(same as above)	Southpaw	ES	Repeat cycle 8 times
(same as above)	Southpaw	FS	Repeat cycle 32 times
AEROJUMP			
EXERCISE	**LENGTH OF TIME**		
Side-Under (FAST)	60 seconds (then rest for 30 seconds)		
Side-Under (FAST)	60 seconds (then rest for 30 seconds)		
Side-Under (FAST)	60 seconds		
AEROSCULPT			
EXERCISE	**LENGTH OF TIME**		
Slow Aero Shuffle	30 seconds (then rest for 30 seconds)		
Slow Aero Shuffle	30 seconds (then rest for 30 seconds)		
Slow Aero Shuffle	30 seconds		

THE SLEEKIFY 5-MINUTE COOLDOWN			
Before you start, catch your breath by walking in place or side to side for 1 minute, or until your heart rate comes down.			
STRETCH	**LENGTH OF TIME/ REPETITIONS**		
Standing Tilt	Repeat twice to each side (hold each portion for 10 seconds)		
Back Bend/Forward Bend	Repeat 4 times back and forth (hold each portion for 10 seconds)		
Biceps-Forearm Stretch	Perform once with each arm (hold each stretch for 10 seconds)		
Shoulder-Triceps Stretch	Perform once with each arm (hold each stretch for 10 seconds)		
Sprinter's Calf Stretch	Perform the stretch 4 times with each leg for 10 seconds each time		
Kneeling Quad Stretch	Perform the stretch twice with each leg for 10 seconds		
Knee Hug	Perform the stretch once for 10 seconds		
Lying Hip-Glute Stretch	Perform the stretch twice with each leg for 10 seconds		
Hip Flexor Stretch	Perform the stretch once with each leg for 10 seconds		

NEW AEROJUMP MOVES

SIDE-UNDER

This variation allows you to alternate between doing the basic jump and swinging the rope along the sides of your body like a propeller so that you don't have to jump over it. It may not seem as intense, but it's designed to improve the coordination between your upper and lower body. The side perk is that it also improves the muscle tone throughout your upper body.

START POSITION: Start by holding the rope at both ends—your arms should be down at your sides, palms facing forward. Step forward so that the middle of the rope is right behind your heels.

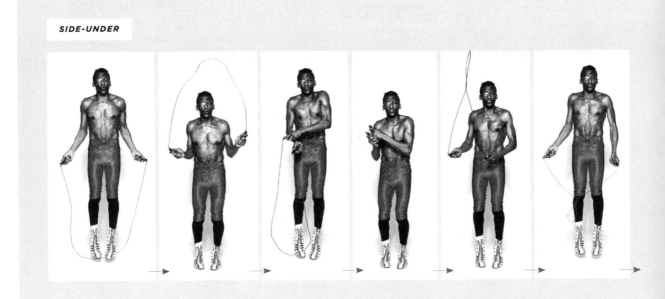

SIDE-UNDER

THE MOVE:

1. Keeping your hands close to your body, begin turning the rope forward, rotating only from your wrists. Once the rope comes down toward your feet, jump over the rope and land on the balls of your feet.

2. As you swing the rope, squat down a few inches as you simultaneously bring your left hand over to your right hand—the rope should swing along the right side of your body.

3. As the rope rises up behind you, bring your left hand back to the starting position, keeping your left hand at waist level as it moves across your body. As the rope lowers toward your feet, jump up to allow the rope to pass underneath you.

4. As you swing the rope, squat down a few inches as you simultaneously bring your right hand over to your left hand—the rope should swing along the left side of your body.

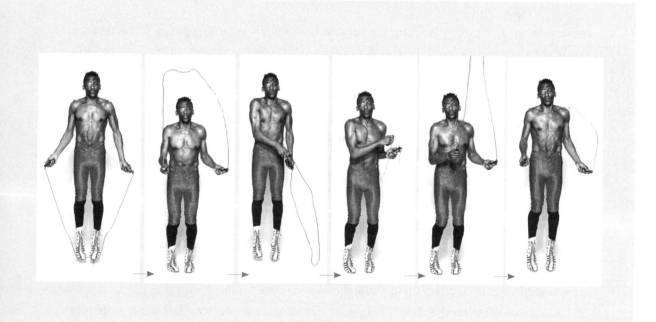

5. As the rope rises up behind you, bring your right hand back to the starting position, keeping your right hand at waist level as you go. As the rope lowers toward your feet, jump up to allow the rope to pass underneath you.

6. Keep alternating from left to right for the duration of the exercise.

Aero-Tip

- Even though you're not technically jumping over the rope two-thirds of the time, you should still be moving at the same tempo as the basic jump—138 jumps per minute.

SIDE-UNDER (FAST)

This advanced variation is exactly the same as a regular side-under from Week Two—only much faster. By raising your tempo to at least 152 jumps per minute—instead of the usual 138—your coordination will improve dramatically, as well as your aerobic conditioning.

START POSITION: Start by holding the rope at both ends—your arms should be down at your sides, palms facing forward. Step forward so that the middle of the rope is right behind your heels.

THE MOVE:

1. Keeping your hands close to your body, begin turning the rope forward, rotating only from your wrists. Once the rope comes down toward your feet, jump over the rope and land on the balls of your feet.

2. As you swing the rope, bring your left hand over to your right hand—the rope should swing along the right side of your body.

3. As the rope rises up behind you, bring your left hand back to the starting position, keeping your left hand at waist level as it moves across your body. As the rope lowers toward your feet, jump up to allow the rope to pass underneath you.

4. As you swing the rope, bring your right hand over to your left hand—the rope should swing along the left side of your body.

5.   As the rope rises up behind you, bring your right hand back to the starting position, keeping your right hand at waist level as you go. As the rope lowers toward your feet, jump up to allow the rope to pass underneath you.

6.   Keep alternating from left to right for the duration of the exercise.

Aero-Tip

- If a regular side-under feels like running to you, then this variation should feel like you're doing a full-out sprint. In other words, if you're not putting everything you have into it, you're not pushing yourself as hard as you should be.

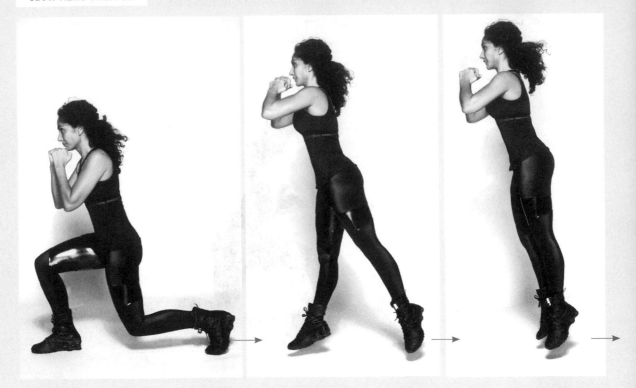

NEW AEROSCULPT MOVES

SLOW AERO SHUFFLE

START POSITION: Stand straight with your feet shoulder width apart, right foot forward and left foot back, fists up by the sides of your face.

THE MOVE: Squat down until your butt is in line with your knees, then quickly jump up so that your feet come a few inches off the floor. While in midair, switch foot positions by bringing your left foot forward and your right foot back. Land on the balls of your

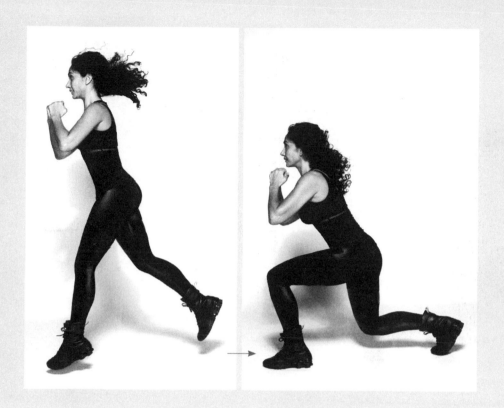

feet, then immediately squat and jump up once more—this time switching foot positions by bringing your right foot forward and left foot back.

Continue switching from right foot forward to left foot forward for the entire exercise.

Aero-Tip

- Keep your quadriceps, glutes, calves, and core muscles flexed the entire time.

Past Aero-Moves to Expect

AEROBOX

- Jab
- Power Punch
- Uppercut
- Hook

AEROJUMP

- (none)

AEROSCULPT

- (none)

New Aero-Moves You Need to Know

AEROBOX

- (none)

AEROJUMP

- Double Under (8-count)
- Double Under (4-count)

AEROSCULPT

- Knee Touch Plio-Jump Squat
- Warrior Squat

THE PROGRAM (DAYS 11, 12, AND 13)

THE SLEEKIFY THREE-MINUTE WARM-UP	
Upper Body	
EXERCISE/STRETCH	**LENGTH OF TIME/REPETITIONS**
Standing Tilt	Repeat 4 times to each side (hold each portion for 5 seconds)
Back Bend/Forward Bend	Repeat 4 times to each side (hold each portion for 5 seconds)
Biceps-Forearm Stretch	Perform once with each arm (hold each stretch for 5 seconds)
Shoulder-Triceps Stretch	Perform once with each arm (hold each stretch for 4–5 seconds)
Lower Body	
Squat Stretch	Perform the stretch once for 10 seconds
Ankle Circles	Perform the move once with each leg for 10 seconds
Standing Calf Raise	Perform the exercise for 30 seconds
Jog (or Jump) in Place	Do for 30 seconds
Tri Jumping Jacks	Perform the 3-part move once for a total of 30 seconds (each variation for 10 seconds)

ROUND ONE

AEROBOX			
TYPE OF PUNCH	**POSITION**	**SPEED**	**DURATION**
(Four 3-move combos) Left Jab, Left Jab, Power Right Power Left, Power Right, Left Hook Power Right, Power Left, Power Right Left Uppercut, Power Right, Left Hook	Orthodox	ES	Repeat cycle 8 times
(same as above)	Orthodox	FS	Repeat cycle 8 times—rest for 4 seconds in between each cycle
(same as above)	Orthodox	FS	Repeat cycle 32 times—no rest in between

(Four 3-move combos) Right Jab, Right Jab, Power Left Power Right, Power Left, Right Hook Power Left, Power Right, Power Left Right Uppercut, Power Left, Right Hook	Southpaw	ES	Repeat cycle 8 times
(same as above)	Southpaw	FS	Repeat cycle 8 times—rest for 4 seconds in between each cycle
(same as above)	Southpaw	FS	Repeat cycle 32 times—no rest in between

AEROJUMP			
EXERCISE	**LENGTH OF TIME**		
Double Under	180 seconds		

AEROSCULPT			
EXERCISE	**LENGTH OF TIME/ REPETITIONS**		
Knee Touch Plio-Jump Squat	Do 16 squats (then rest 30–45 seconds)		
Repeat this exercise 4 times for a total of 64 squats			

ROUND TWO

AEROBOX			
TYPE OF PUNCH	**POSITION**	**SPEED**	**DURATION**
(Four 3-move combos) Left Jab, Left Jab, Left Jab Right Uppercut, Left Hook, Power Right Power Left, Left Hook, Power Right Left Uppercut, Left Hook, Power Right	Orthodox	ES	Repeat cycle 8 times
(same as above)	Orthodox	FS	Repeat cycle 8 times—rest for 4 seconds in between each cycle
(same as above)	Orthodox	FS	Repeat cycle 32 times—no rest in between

(Four 3-move combos) Right Jab, Right Jab, Right Jab Left Uppercut, Right Hook, Power Left Power Right, Right Hook, Power Left Right Uppercut, Right Hook, Power Left	Southpaw	ES	Repeat cycle 8 times
(same as above)	Southpaw	FS	Repeat cycle 8 times—rest for 4 seconds in between each cycle
(same as above)	Southpaw	FS	Repeat cycle 32 times—no rest in between

AEROJUMP			
EXERCISE	**LENGTH OF TIME**		
Double Under	180 seconds		

AEROSCULPT			
EXERCISE	**LENGTH OF TIME/ REPETITIONS**		
Knee Touch Plio-Jump Squat	Do 16 squats (then rest 30–45 seconds)		
Repeat this exercise 4 times for a total of 64 squats			

ROUND THREE

AEROBOX			
TYPE OF PUNCH	**POSITION**	**SPEED**	**DURATION**
(24-move combo—This series of punches may look complex, but you're actually doing the same 8-move Orthodox combos from Rounds One and Two back-to-back.) Left Jab, Left Jab, Power Right, Power Left, Power Right, Left Hook, Power Right, Power Left, Power Right, Left Uppercut, Power Right, Left Hook, Left Jab, Left Jab, Left Jab, Right Uppercut, Left Hook, Power Right, Power Left, Left Hook, Power Right, Left Uppercut, Left Hook, Power Right	Orthodox	ES	Repeat cycle 8 times
(same as above)	Orthodox	FS	Repeat cycle 8 times—rest for 4 seconds in between each cycle

(same as above)	Orthodox	FS	Repeat cycle 32 times—no rest in between
(24-move combo—This series of punches may look complex, but you're actually doing the same 8-move Southpaw combos from Rounds One and Two back-to-back.) Right Jab, Right Jab, Power Left, Power Right, Power Left, Right Hook, Power Left, Power Right, Power Left, Right Upper-cut, Power Left, Right Hook, Right Jab, Right Jab, Right Jab, Left Uppercut, Right Hook, Power Left, Power Right, Right Hook, Power Left, Right Upper-cut, Right Hook, Power Left	Southpaw	ES	Repeat cycle 8 times
(same as above)	Southpaw	FS	Repeat cycle 8 times—rest for 4 seconds in between each cycle
(same as above)	Southpaw	FS	Repeat cycle 32 times—no rest in between

AEROJUMP			
EXERCISE	**LENGTH OF TIME**		
Double Under (4-count)	180 seconds		

AEROSCULPT			
EXERCISE	**LENGTH OF TIME/ REPETITIONS**		
Warrior Squat (strive for a 1/3 pace, taking 1 second to touch your feet and 3 seconds to bring your feet apart)	Do 16 squats (then rest 30–45 sec-onds)		
Warrior Squat (strive for a 1/2 pace, taking 1 second to touch your feet and 2 seconds to bring your feet apart)	Do 32 squats (then rest 30–45 sec-onds); repeat 3 more times for a total of 4 sets (128 squats)		

THE SLEEKIFY 5-MINUTE COOLDOWN			
Before you start, catch your breath by walking in place or side to side for 1 minute, or until your heart rate comes down.			
STRETCH	**LENGTH OF TIME/ REPETITIONS**		
Standing Tilt	Repeat twice to each side (hold each portion for 10 seconds)		
Back Bend/Forward Bend	Repeat 4 times back and forth (hold each portion for 10 seconds)		
Biceps-Forearm Stretch	Perform once with each arm (hold each stretch for 10 seconds)		
Shoulder-Triceps Stretch	Perform once with each arm (hold each stretch for 10 seconds)		
Sprinter's Calf Stretch	Perform the stretch 4 times with each leg for 10 seconds each time		
Kneeling Quad Stretch	Perform the stretch twice with each leg for 10 seconds		
Knee Hug	Perform the stretch once for 10 seconds		
Lying Hip-Glute Stretch	Perform the stretch twice with each leg for 10 seconds		
Hip Flexor Stretch	Perform the stretch once with each leg for 10 seconds		

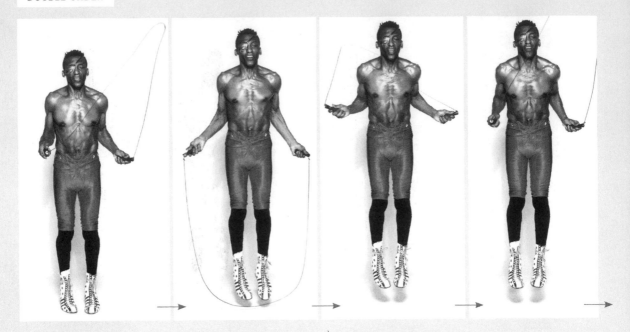

NEW AEROJUMP MOVES

DOUBLE UNDER (8-COUNT)

This variation is the basic jump. The only difference: Jump the rope as you count from 1 to 8 repeatedly. Every time you return to 1, you'll jump slightly higher and quickly turn your wrist so the rope passes not once, but twice below you before you land. Done right, it offers all the benefits of the basic jump, plus improves your anaerobic conditioning, coordination, and speed.

START POSITION: Start by holding the rope at both ends—your arms should be down at your sides, palms facing forward. Step forward so that the middle of the rope is right behind your heels.

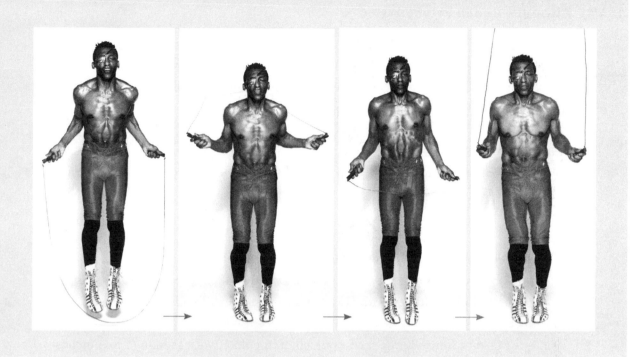

THE MOVE:

1.   Keeping your hands close to your body, begin turning the rope forward, rotating only from your wrists. Once the rope comes down toward your feet, take a tiny hop to allow the rope to pass underneath you. Land on the balls of your feet and repeat for 8 jumps.

2.   After your eighth jump, push yourself off the floor twice as high (2 to 4 inches) and quickly spin the rope faster than usual so that it passes beneath you twice—instead of once—before you land. Land on the balls of your feet and repeat for 7 more jumps.

3.   Continue to alternate between doing 1 double under and 7 basic jumps for the remainder of the exercise.

Aero-Tip

- You may feel like you have to pull your heels back to give the rope enough space to go underneath you twice—try not to! Just jumping a little higher by pushing more off the balls of your feet—and the right effort from your wrists—is all you need.

This variation is a double under, only instead of turning the rope twice every 8 jumps, you'll reduce the time to every 4 jumps. The benefits are the same as the 8-count double under, but it pushes your upper body and cardio even harder by ramping up the intensity.

START POSITION: Start by holding the rope at both ends—your arms should be down at your sides, palms facing forward. Step forward so that the middle of the rope is right behind your heels.

THE MOVE:

1. Keeping your hands close to your body, begin turning the rope forward, rotating only from your wrists. Once the rope comes down toward your feet, take a tiny hop to allow the rope to pass underneath you. Land on the balls of your feet and repeat for 4 jumps.

2. After your fourth jump, push yourself off the floor twice as high (2 to 4 inches) and quickly spin the rope faster than usual so that it passes beneath you twice—instead of once—before you land. Land on the balls of your feet and repeat for 3 more jumps.

3. Continue to alternate between doing 1 double under and 3 basic jumps for the remainder of the exercise.

Aero-Tip

- You may feel like you have to pull your heels back to give the rope enough space to go underneath you twice—try not to! Just jumping a little higher by pushing more off the balls of your feet—and the right effort from your wrists—is all you need.

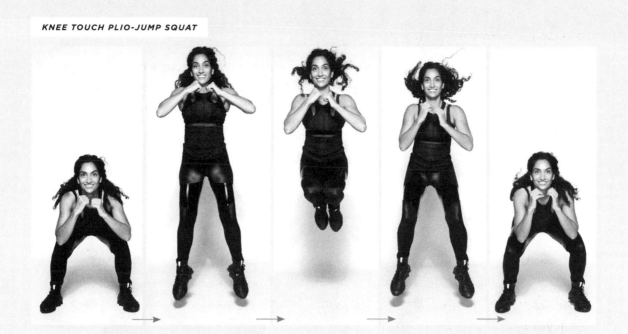

KNEE TOUCH PLIO-JUMP SQUAT

NEW AEROSCULPT MOVES

KNEE TOUCH PLIO-JUMP SQUAT

START POSITION: Stand straight with your legs together, feet slightly wider than shoulder width apart, fists up by the sides of your face.

THE MOVE: Squat down until your butt is in line with your knees, then quickly jump up so that your feet come a few inches off the floor. While in midair, bring your legs together so they touch as you draw your knees up and your feet under you, then quickly spread your legs back out—as you land on the balls of your feet, your feet should be slightly wider than shoulder width apart once more. Continue to squat, jump, and touch/spread your legs for a total of 4 times.

Aero-Tip

- Keep your quadriceps, glutes, calves, and core muscles flexed the entire time.

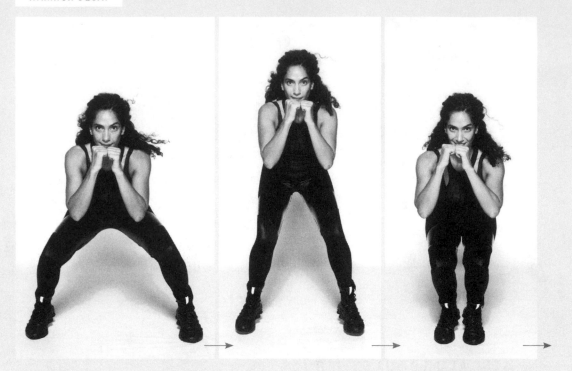

WARRIOR SQUAT

START POSITION: Stand straight with your legs together, feet wider than shoulder width apart, fists up by the sides of your face.

THE MOVE: Squat down until your butt is in line with your knees, then quickly jump up so that your feet barely come off the floor. Slide your feet toward each other—your feet should feel as if they're skimming along the floor—so your knees touch as you squat down once more. Immediately hop up again so that your feet barely come off the floor, but this time, slide your feet apart so that you end up with your feet wider than shoulder width apart as you squat back down. Repeat this cycle 8 times.

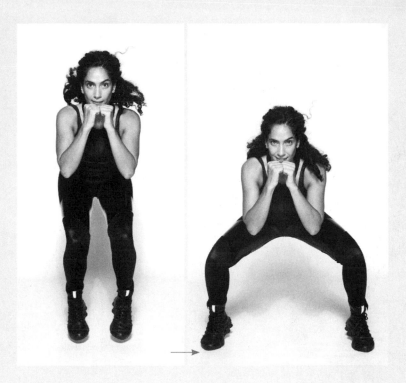

Aero-Tips

- Your knees should remain bent throughout the movement.
- Keep your quadriceps, glutes, calves, and core muscles flexed the entire time.

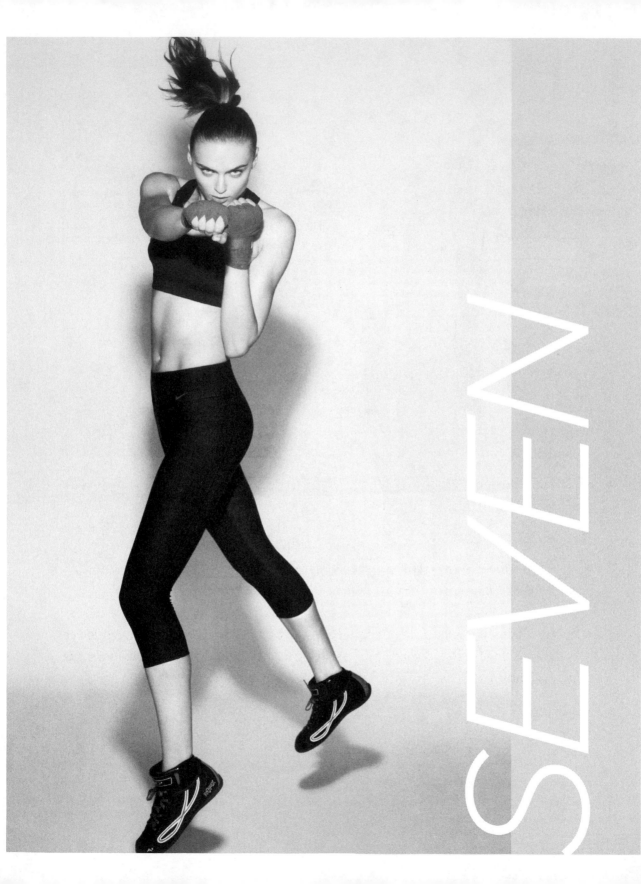

WEEK THREE

FOR WEEK THREE, YOU'LL CONTINUE TO BEGIN EACH WORKOUT AND USE IT for a total of three straight days before moving on to the next workout.

After the six-day cycle is over, you'll rest on the seventh day before moving on to Week Four. Or you can add a seventh workout by either repeating the last day of the routine you've previously finished or starting whichever routine you'll be doing the following week a day earlier.

As you move from exercise to exercise within each round, you will rest for only as long as it takes you to get into position. However, between rounds, you have the choice of either resting for sixty seconds before starting the next round or keeping the intensity high by immediately jumping into the next round without any rest.

Past Aero-Moves to Expect

AEROBOX

- Jab
- Power Punch
- Uppercut
- Hook

AEROJUMP

- Double Under (4-count)

AEROSCULPT

- (none)

New Aero-Moves You Need to Know

AEROBOX

- (none)

AEROJUMP

- Boxer Skip
- Crossover Hold

AEROSCULPT

- Aerofly (Level One)

THE PROGRAM (DAYS 15, 16, AND 17)

THE SLEEKIFY 3-MINUTE WARM-UP	
Upper Body	
EXERCISE/STRETCH	LENGTH OF TIME/REPETITIONS
Standing Tilt	Repeat 4 times to each side (hold each portion for 5 seconds)
Back Bend/Forward Bend	Repeat 4 times to each side (hold each portion for 5 seconds)
Biceps-Forearm Stretch	Perform once with each arm (hold each stretch for 5 seconds)
Shoulder-Triceps Stretch	Perform once with each arm (hold each stretch for 4–5 seconds)
Lower Body	
Squat Stretch	Perform the stretch once for 10 seconds
Ankle Circles	Perform the move once with each leg for 10 seconds
Standing Calf Raise	Perform the exercise for 30 seconds
Jog (or Jump) in Place	Do for 30 seconds
Tri Jumping Jacks	Perform the 3-part move once for a total of 30 seconds (each variation for 10 seconds)

ROUND ONE

AEROBOX			
TYPE OF PUNCH	POSITION	SPEED	DURATION
(8-move combo) Left Jab, Left Jab, Power Right, Right Jab, Power Left, Power Right, Left Hook, Right Hook	Pyramid	FS	Repeat cycle 4 times—rest for 4 seconds in between each cycle
(same as above)	Pyramid	FS	Repeat cycle 4 times—rest for 4 seconds in between each cycle
(same as above)	Pyramid	FS	Repeat cycle 32 times—no rest in between
(8-move combo) Right Jab, Right Jab, Power Left, Left Jab, Power Right, Power Left, Right Hook, Left Hook	Pyramid	ES	Repeat cycle 4 times—rest for 4 seconds in between each cycle
(same as above)	Pyramid	FS	Repeat cycle 4 times—rest for 4 seconds in between each cycle

| (same as above) | Pyramid | FS | Repeat cycle 32 times—no rest in between |

AEROJUMP			
EXERCISE	**LENGTH OF TIME**		
Boxer Skip	180 seconds		
Crossover Holds	60 seconds		
Double Under (4-count)	180 seconds		

AEROSCULPT			
EXERCISE	**LENGTH OF TIME/ REPETITIONS**		
Aerofly (Level One) standing on left leg	64 reps		
Aerofly (Level One) standing on right leg	64 reps		

ROUND TWO

AEROBOX			
TYPE OF PUNCH	**POSITION**	**SPEED**	**DURATION**
(8-move combo) Left Jab, Left Jab, Power Right, Power Right, Power Left, Power Right, Left Hook, Right Hook	Orthodox	ES	Repeat cycle 16 times
(same as above)	Orthodox	FS	Repeat cycle 8 times—rest for 4 seconds in between each cycle
(same as above)	Orthodox	FS	Do two cycles back-to-back (for a total of 16 punches). Rest for 4 seconds. Repeat the entire 16-punch/ 4-second rest cycle 8 times
(same as above)	Orthodox	FS	Repeat cycle 32 times—no rest in between

AEROJUMP			
EXERCISE	**LENGTH OF TIME**		
Boxer Skip	180 seconds		
Crossover Holds	60 seconds		
Double Under (4-count)	180 seconds		

AEROSCULPT		
EXERCISE	**LENGTH OF TIME/ REPETITIONS**	
Aerofly (Level One) standing on left leg	64 reps	
Aerofly (Level One) standing on right leg	64 reps	

ROUND THREE

AEROBOX			
TYPE OF PUNCH	**POSITION**	**SPEED**	**DURATION**
(8-move combo) Right Jab, Right Jab, Power Left, Power Left, Power Right, Power Left, Right Hook, Left Hook	Southpaw	ES	Repeat cycle 16 times
(same as above)	Southpaw	FS	Repeat cycle 8 times—rest for 4 seconds in between each cycle
(same as above)	Southpaw	FS	Do two cycles back-to-back (for a total of 16 punches). Rest for 4 seconds. Repeat the entire 16-punch/4-second rest cycle 8 times
(same as above)	Southpaw	FS	Repeat cycle 32 times—no rest in between

AEROJUMP			
EXERCISE	**LENGTH OF TIME**		
Boxer Skip	180 seconds		
Crossover Holds	60 seconds		
Double Under (1-count)	180 seconds		

AEROSCULPT			
EXERCISE	**LENGTH OF TIME/ REPETITIONS**		
Aerofly (Level One) standing on left leg	64 reps		
Aerofly (Level One) standing on right leg	64 reps		

THE SLEEKIFY 5-MINUTE COOLDOWN

Before you start, catch your breath by walking in place or side to side for 1 minute, or until your heart rate comes down.

STRETCH	LENGTH OF TIME/ REPETITIONS		
Standing Tilt	Repeat twice to each side (hold each portion for 10 seconds)		
Back Bend/Forward Bend	Repeat 4 times back and forth (hold each portion for 10 seconds)		
Biceps-Forearm Stretch	Perform once with each arm (hold each stretch for 10 seconds)		
Shoulder-Triceps Stretch	Perform once with each arm (hold each stretch for 10 seconds)		
Sprinter's Calf Stretch	Perform the stretch 4 times with each leg for 10 seconds each time		
Kneeling Quad Stretch	Perform the stretch twice with each leg for 10 seconds		
Knee Hug	Perform the stretch once for 10 seconds		
Lying Hip-Glute Stretch	Perform the stretch twice with each leg for 10 seconds		
Hip Flexor Stretch	Perform the stretch once with each leg for 10 seconds		

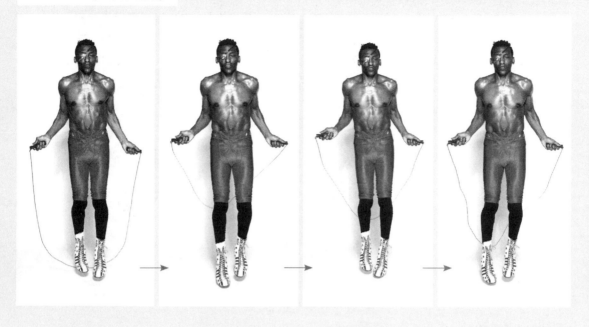

NEW AEROJUMP MOVES

BOXER SKIP

This classic boxing maneuver—which may feel like a one-leg skip—actually has you shifting your weight from one foot to the other. This low-intensity drill helps improve your coordination for other jumps, while offering your muscles a form of recovery to give them a break during harder portions of the workout.

START POSITION: Start by holding the rope at both ends—your arms should be down at your sides, palms facing forward. Step forward so that the middle of the rope is right behind your heels.

THE MOVE:

1.   Keeping your hands close to your body, begin turning the rope forward, rotating only from your wrists. Once the rope comes down toward your feet, take a tiny hop to allow the rope to pass underneath you.

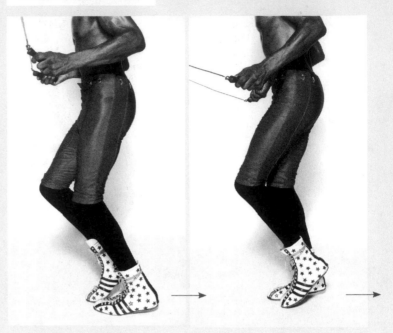

BOXER SKIP (SIDE VIEW)

2. As you land, let your right knee come up in front of you slightly so that you land on the ball of your left foot—your right toes will just touch the floor. Repeat for four jumps.

3. Jump back up to let the rope pass underneath again, only this time, let your left knee come up in front of you slightly so that you land on the ball of your right foot—your left toes will just touch the floor. Repeat for eight jumps.

4. Repeat steps 1 and 2, only this time, do four jumps per leg.

5. Repeat steps 2 and 3, only this time, do two jumps per leg.

6. Repeat steps 2 and 3, only this time, do one jump per leg.

7. Continue to alternate from shifting your weight onto your left foot (for one jump) to your right foot (for one jump) for the duration of the exercise.

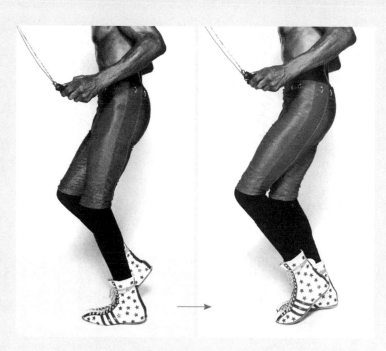

Acro-Tips

- With the boxer skip, it's a very subtle shifting of your weight from one foot to the other. Your shoulder weight is going over to side to side. When you go to the left, your right knee comes up; when you go to the right, your left knee comes up.

- As you slightly shift your weight to the right, drop your right heel lower to the ground—your left heel should be higher—and vice versa when shifting your weight onto your left leg.

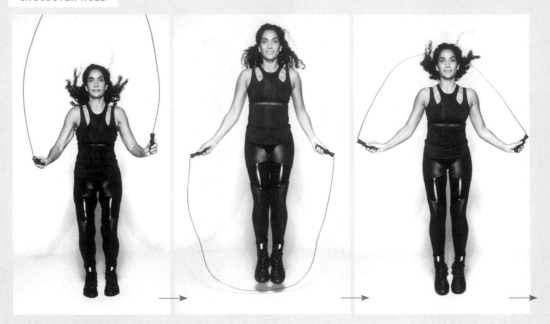

CROSSOVER HOLD

CROSSOVER HOLD

This advanced technique is simply a basic skip, only half the time, you'll have your arms crossed in front of you. It's a change-up that will enhance your dexterity while helping to tone your chest and shoulder muscles at the same time.

START POSITION: Start by holding the rope at both ends—your arms should be down at your sides, palms facing forward. Step forward so that the middle of the rope is right behind your heels.

THE MOVE:

1.   Keeping your hands close to your body, begin turning the rope forward, rotating only from your wrists. Once the rope comes down toward your feet, take a tiny hop to allow the rope to pass underneath you. Land on the balls of your feet and repeat for eight jumps.

2.   As the rope is in the air, cross your arms at your elbows in front of your body. Your hands should end up wider than and below your waist, with your left hand positioned along the right side of your body and your right hand positioned along the left side of your body.

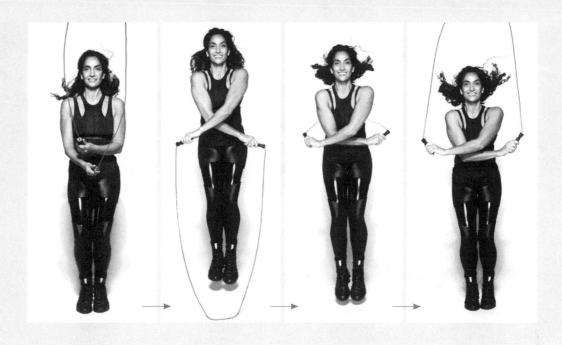

3.   Land on the balls of your feet and repeat, keeping your arms crossed in front of you, for eight more jumps.

4.   As the rope comes back down in front of you, uncross your arms and bring your hands back to the start position. Continue to alternate between doing eight basic jumps, then doing eight crossovers for the remainder of the exercise.

Aero-Tips

- With your arms crossed, you'll find you'll feel the move more in your wrists. That's because being crossed prevents your arms from contributing as much work, leaving your wrists to handle more of the effort of turning the rope.

- It may feel strange at first to jump over the rope when your hands are crossed in front of you. For some people, it feels almost like a trick of the eyes, making you believe there's not enough rope to pass below your feet. But don't worry, and break that fear—if your form is solid, the rope will always be open when you're ready to jump over it.

NEW AEROSCULPT MOVES

AEROFLY (LEVEL ONE)

START POSITION: Stand straight with your legs together and your arms hanging straight down at your sides. Bend your knees slightly as you bend forward at the waist and touch the floor with your fingertips. (If you're not that flexible, place a sturdy box about 2 to 4 inches high on the floor—or even a pair of light hand weights stood up on end—to rest your fingertips on instead.) Finally, bend your left leg behind you at about a 90-degree angle, left foot suspended a few inches off the floor.

THE MOVE: Keeping your left leg bent behind you, press yourself upward by pushing your right foot into the floor. As you rise, simultaneously sweep your arms out to your sides—like a pair of wings. Lower yourself back down into the start position and repeat.

Perform the exercise for as many repetitions as required, then switch leg positions and repeat the exercise—balancing on your left foot with your right foot bent behind you, fingertips touching the floor.

Aero-Tips

- Keep your quadriceps, glutes, calves, and core muscles flexed the entire time.
- Keep your head down as you go—raising your head too far up may strain your neck muscles.

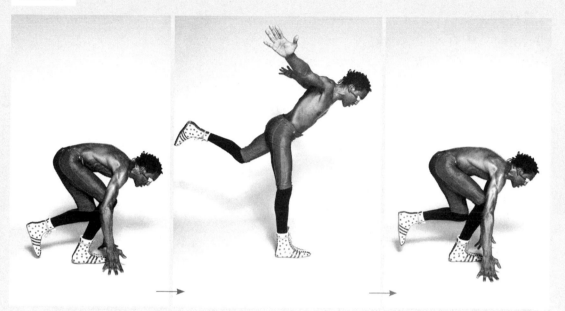

AEROFLY

Past Aero-Moves to Expect

AEROBOX

- Jab
- Power Punch
- Uppercut
- Hook
- Lateral Slip

AEROJUMP

- Boxer Skip
- Double Under

AEROSCULPT

- (none)

New Aero-Moves You Need to Know

AEROBOX

- Lateral Slip to Right
- Lateral Slip to Left

AEROJUMP

- Crossover Single Out

AEROSCULPT

- Aerofly (Level Two—Toe Lift)
- Aerofly (Level Three—Single-Leg Hop)

THE PROGRAM (DAYS 18, 19, AND 20)

THE SLEEKIFY 3-MINUTE WARM-UP	
Upper Body	
EXERCISE/STRETCH	**LENGTH OF TIME/REPETITIONS**
Standing Tilt	Repeat 4 times to each side (hold each portion for 5 seconds)
Back Bend/Forward Bend	Repeat 4 times to each side (hold each portion for 5 seconds)
Biceps-Forearm Stretch	Perform once with each arm (hold each stretch for 5 seconds)
Shoulder-Triceps Stretch	Perform once with each arm (hold each stretch for 4–5 seconds)
Lower Body	
Squat Stretch	Perform the stretch once for 10 seconds
Ankle Circles	Perform the move once with each leg for 10 seconds
Standing Calf Raise	Perform the exercise for 30 seconds
Jog (or Jump) in Place	Do for 30 seconds
Tri Jumping Jacks	Perform the 3-part move once for a total of 30 seconds (each variation for 10 seconds)

ROUND ONE

AEROBOX			
TYPE OF PUNCH	**POSITION**	**SPEED**	**DURATION**
(8-move combo) Left Uppercut, Power Right, Left Hook, Power Right, Lateral Slip to Right, Left Jab, Left Jab, Power Right	Pyramid	DS	Repeat cycle 8 times
(same as above)	Pyramid	ES	Repeat cycle 16 times
(same as above)	Pyramid	ΓS	Repeat cycle 8 times—rest for 4 seconds in between each cycle
(same as above)	Pyramid	FS	Do two cycles back-to-back (for a total of 16 punches). Rest for 4 seconds. Repeat the entire 16-punch/4-second rest cycle 8 times
(same as above)	Pyramid	FS	Repeat cycle 32 times—no rest in between

(8-move combo) Right Uppercut, Power Left, Right Hook, Power Left, Lateral Slip to Left, Right Jab, Right Jab, Power Left	Pyramid	DS	Repeat cycle 8 times
(same as above)	Pyramid	ES	Repeat cycle 16 times
(same as above)	Pyramid	FS	Repeat cycle 8 times—rest for 4 seconds in between each cycle
(same as above)	Pyramid	FS	Do 2 cycles back-to-back (for a total of 16 punches). Rest for 4 seconds. Repeat the entire 16-punch/4-second rest cycle 8 times
(same as above)	Pyramid	FS	Repeat cycle 32 times—no rest in between

AEROJUMP			
EXERCISE	**LENGTH OF TIME**		
Boxer Skip	60 seconds		
Crossovers Single Out	60 seconds		
Double Under	120 seconds		

AEROSCULPT			
EXERCISE	**LENGTH OF TIME/ REPETITIONS**		
Aerofly (Level Two—Toe Lift) standing on left leg	64 reps		
Aerofly (Level Two—Toe Lift) standing on right leg	64 reps		

ROUND TWO

AEROBOX			
TYPE OF PUNCH	**POSITION**	**SPEED**	**DURATION**
(8-move combo) Left Uppercut, Power Right, Left Hook, Power Right, Lateral Slip to Right, Left Jab, Left Jab, Power Right	Orthodox	DS	Repeat cycle 8 times
(same as above)	Orthodox	ES	Repeat cycle 16 times

(same as above)	Orthodox	FS	Repeat cycle 8 times—rest for 4 seconds in between each cycle
(same as above)	Orthodox	FS	Do 2 cycles back-to-back (for a total of 16 punches). Rest for 4 seconds. Repeat the entire 16-punch/4-second rest cycle 8 times
(same as above)	Orthodox	FS	Repeat cycle 32 times—no rest in between

AEROJUMP			
EXERCISE	LENGTH OF TIME		
Boxer Skip	60 seconds		
Crossovers Single Out	60 seconds		
Double Under	120 seconds		

AEROSCULPT			
EXERCISE	LENGTH OF TIME/REPETITIONS		
Aerofly (Level Two—Toe Lift) standing on left leg	64 reps		
Aerofly (Level Two—Toe Lift) standing on right leg	64 reps		

ROUND THREE

AEROBOX			
TYPE OF PUNCH	POSITION	SPEED	DURATION
(8-move combo) Right Uppercut, Power Left, Right Hook, Power Left, Lateral Slip to Left, Right Jab, Right Jab, Power Left	Southpaw	DS	Repeat cycle 8 times
(same as above)	Southpaw	ES	Repeat cycle 16 times
(same as above)	Southpaw	FS	Repeat cycle 8 times—rest for 4 seconds in between each cycle

(same as above)	Southpaw	FS	Do 2 cycles back-to-back (for a total of 16 punches). Rest for 4 seconds. Repeat the entire 16-punch/ 4-second rest cycle 8 times
(same as above)	Southpaw	FS	Repeat cycle 32 times—no rest in between

AEROJUMP			
EXERCISE	**LENGTH OF TIME**		
Boxer Skip	60 seconds		
Crossovers Single Out	60 seconds		
Double Under (Instead of doing a double under every 8 jumps, do 2 consecutive double unders back-to-back every 16 jumps.)	120 seconds		

AEROSCULPT			
EXERCISE	**LENGTH OF TIME/ REPETITIONS**		
Aerofly (Level Three— Single-Leg Hop) standing on left leg	64 reps		
Aerofly (Level Three— Single-Leg Hop) standing on right leg	64 reps		

THE SLEEKIFY 5-MINUTE COOLDOWN			
Before you start, catch your breath by walking in place or side to side for 1 minute, or until your heart rate comes down.			
STRETCH	**LENGTH OF TIME/ REPETITIONS**		
Standing Tilt	Repeat twice to each side (hold each portion for 10 seconds)		
Back Bend/Forward Bend	Repeat 4 times back and forth (hold each portion for 10 seconds)		
Biceps-Forearm Stretch	Perform once with each arm (hold each stretch for 10 seconds)		

Shoulder-Triceps Stretch	Perform once with each arm (hold each stretch for 10 seconds)		
Sprinter's Calf Stretch	Perform the stretch 4 times with each leg for 10 seconds each time		
Kneeling Quad Stretch	Perform the stretch twice with each leg for 10 seconds		
Knee Hug	Perform the stretch once for 10 seconds		
Lying Hip-Glute Stretch	Perform the stretch twice with each leg for 10 seconds		
Hip Flexor Stretch	Perform the stretch once with each leg for 10 seconds		

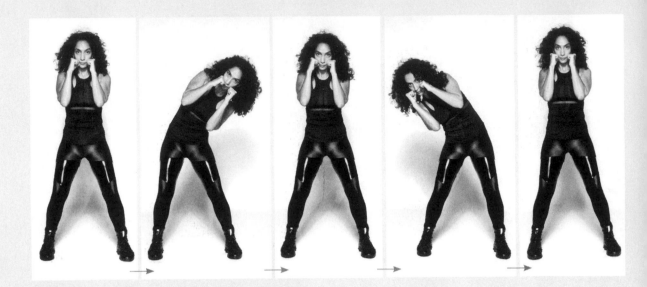

NEW AEROBOX MOVES

LATERAL SLIP

START POSITION: Start in pyramid position with your feet slightly wider than shoulder width apart, toes pointing forward, knees slightly bent (but muscles flexed). Your fists should be up along the sides of your face, palms facing in.

THE MOVE: To do it to the left, bend slightly at the waist and lean forward and to the left so that your left shoulder drops lower than your right shoulder. To do it to the right, bend slightly at the waist and lean forward and to the right so that your right shoulder drops lower than your left shoulder.

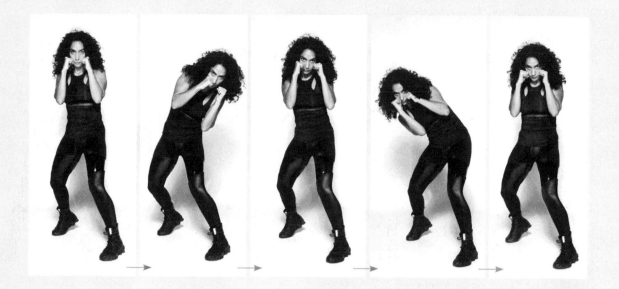

Aero-Tips

- Whichever side you move to, your head should remain straight with your fists up by the sides of your face.
- Don't just lean to each side. In boxing, this move is used to cut the distance between you and your opponent, so moving forward and to the side simultaneously is your goal.

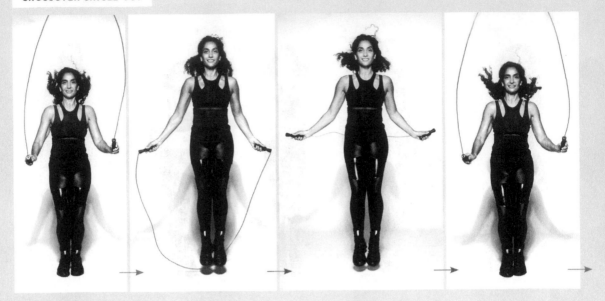

NEW AEROJUMP MOVES

CROSSOVER SINGLE OUT

This advanced technique has you alternating between a basic jump and a crossover every jump. The benefits are the same as the crossover hold, but the intensity picks up a step.

START POSITION: Start by holding the rope at both ends—your arms should be down at your sides, palms facing forward. Step forward so that the middle of the rope is right behind your heels.

THE MOVE:

1.   Keeping your hands close to your body, begin turning the rope forward, rotating only from your wrists. Once the rope comes down toward your feet, take a tiny hop to allow the rope to pass underneath you. Land on the balls of your feet and repeat a few times just to help get your rhythm down.

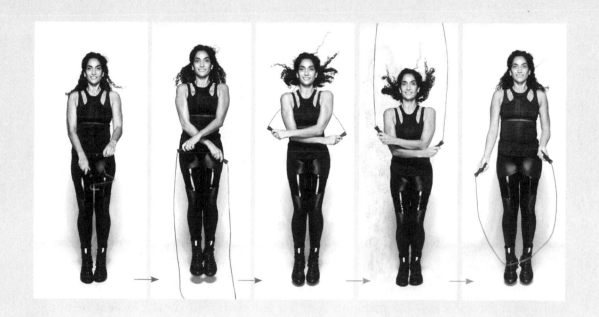

2.   As the rope is in the air, quickly cross your arms at your elbows in front of your body. Your hands should end up wider than and below your waist, left hand along the right side of your body and right hand along the left side.

3.   Jump up to let the rope pass below you, then immediately uncross your arms and bring your hands back to the start position. Jump up to let the rope pass below you once more and repeat. Continue to alternate between doing one basic jump and one crossover for the remainder of the exercise.

Aero-Tips

- With your arms crossed, you'll find you feel the move more in your wrists. That's because being crossed prevents your arms from contributing as much work, leaving your wrists to handle more of the effort of turning the rope.

- A lot of people will cross their hands in, then panic and pull their hands out too quickly. This will mess up your tempo and can cause you to tangle up in the rope. The trick is to bring your hands in—and pull your hands back out—at the same pace.

NEW AEROSCULPT MOVES

AEROFLY (LEVEL TWO—TOE LIFT)

START POSITION: Same as Aerofly (Level One)

THE MOVE: Keeping your left leg bent behind you, press yourself upward by pushing your right foot into the floor. As you rise, simultaneously sweep your arms out to your sides—like a pair of wings. At the very top of the move, lift the toes of your right foot upward as far as you can before lowering yourself back down into the start position.

Perform the exercise for as many repetitions as required, then switch leg positions and repeat the exercise—balancing on your left foot with your right foot bent behind you, fingertips touching the floor.

Aero-Tips

- Keep your quadriceps, glutes, calves, and core muscles flexed the entire time.
- Keep your head down as you go—raising your head too far up may strain your neck muscles.

AEROFLY—TOE LIFT

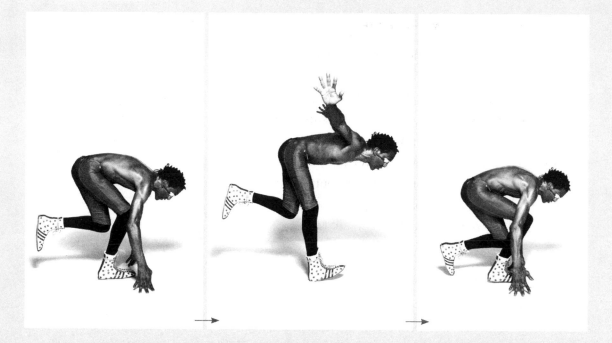

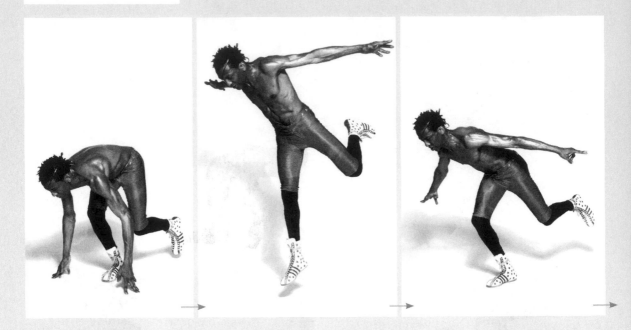

AEROFLY (LEVEL THREE—SINGLE-LEG HOP)

START POSITION: Same as Aerofly (Level One)

THE MOVE: Keeping your left leg bent behind you, forcefully press yourself upward so that you pop off the floor. In midair, quickly sweep your arms out to the sides—like a pair of wings—then sweep them back in front of you so that your fingertips return to the start position.

As you reverse the motion and land, you should come down on the ball of your foot, then roll down to your heel. Don't come down flat-footed, which will make your muscles work less and put more stress on your knee.

The moment you land—right foot on the floor, fingertips touching the floor—

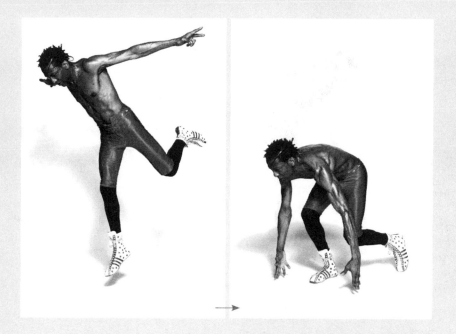

immediately squat down and repeat. Throughout the entire exercise, your left leg should stay bent with your left foot off the floor.

Perform the exercise for as many repetitions as required, then switch leg positions and repeat the exercise—balancing on your left foot with your right leg bent behind you, fingertips touching the floor.

Aero-Tip

- Keep your quadriceps, glutes, calves, and core muscles flexed the entire time.

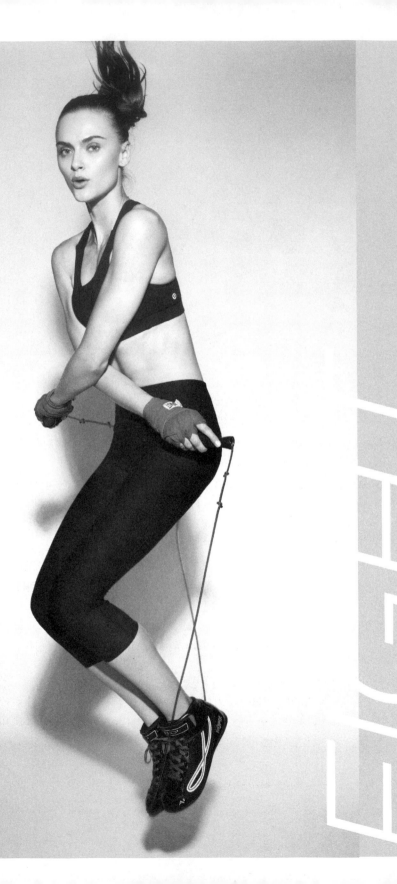

EIGHT

WEEK FOUR

FOR THE FINAL WEEK OF SLEEKIFY, YOU'LL CONTINUE TO BEGIN EACH WORK-out and use it for a total of three straight days before moving on to the next workout. After the six-day cycle is over, you'll either rest on the seventh day or you can add a seventh workout by repeating the last day of the routine.

As you move from exercise to exercise within each round, you will rest for only as long as it takes you to get into position. However, between rounds, you have the choice of either resting for 30 to 60 seconds before starting the next round or keeping the intensity high by immediately jumping into the next round without any rest.

The Changes to the Program—and Why

The first thing you'll notice is a new warm-up that adds a series of punch combos in between the Stim Stretches you've been using during the previous three weeks. That's because this final week is the most intense of the four, and your muscles need to be thoroughly warm and pliable from head to toe before you jump in and perform the program.

You'll also notice a series of new Aerobox moves in the final three-day workout—

moves such as the Ali Shuffle and the Duran Drop. These new moves are a combination of some of my favorite—and what I think are some of the most effective—boxing moves you can practice. These moves are maneuvers that some of the most incredible fighters in the sport once did in the ring, along with others that I've learned over the years working with some of the world's greatest trainers.

Other moves you'll learn in this final week are ones I discovered on my own—alone in the ring. Moves that were bred out of necessity while making things up on the fly during a fight. Moves that I began incorporating into my training until they became effortless. You need patience and repetition to execute these new Aerobox moves seamlessly and make them your own.

Finally, you'll notice the longer duration of combos, some of which will have you throwing and dodging as many as twenty-four punches in a row. These combinations will take much longer to do as you're learning them, but trust me: Once you're proficient at them, the workouts move very fast, and that's when you'll fly.

All of the other drills that you've worked on over the first three weeks were building up to this moment. Week Four is the closest experience you'll get to stepping into Aerospace and experiencing what it's like to take one of my classes and train with me face-to-face. If you're ready for the challenge, then let's go.

DAYS 22, 23, AND 24

Past Aero-Moves to Expect

AEROBOX

- Jab
- Power Punch
- Uppercut
- Hook
- Lateral Slip

AEROJUMP

- Boxer Skip
- Double Under
- Side-Under (Fast)

AEROSCULPT

- (none)

New Aero-Moves You Need to Know

AEROBOX

- (none)

AEROJUMP

- (none)

AEROSCULPT

- Aerofly (Level Four—Single-Leg Exchange)
- Ankle Touch into Warrior

THE PROGRAM (DAYS 22, 23, AND 24)

NEW WEEK FOUR WARM-UP			
AEROBOX			
TYPE OF PUNCH	POSITION	SPEED	DURATION
(8-move combo) Left Jab, Left Jab, Power Right, Power Right, Power Left, Power Right, Left Hook, Right Hook	Orthodox	ES	Repeat cycle 8 times
(8-move combo) Left Uppercut, Power Right, Left Hook, Power Right, Lateral Slip to Right, Left Jab, Left Jab, Power Right	Orthodox	ES	Repeat cycle 8 times

(16-move combo—just combine the last two combos in one longer combo) Left Jab, Left Jab, Power Right, Power Right, Power Left, Power Right, Left Hook, Right Hook, Left Uppercut, Power Right, Left Hook, Power Right, Lateral Slip to Right, Left Jab, Left Jab, Power Right	Orthodox	ES	Repeat cycle 16 times

Stimulation Stretch for Upper Body

EXERCISE/STRETCH	LENGTH OF TIME/ REPETITIONS		
Standing Tilt	Repeat 4 times to each side (hold each portion for 10 seconds)		
Back Bend/Forward Bend	Repeat 4 times to each side (hold each portion for 10 seconds)		
Biceps-Forearm Stretch	Perform once with each arm (hold each stretch for 8 seconds)		
Shoulder-Triceps Stretch	Perform once with each arm (hold each stretch for 4–5 seconds)		

AEROBOX

TYPE OF PUNCH	POSITION	SPEED	DURATION
(8-move combo) Right Jab, Right Jab, Power Left, Power Left, Power Right, Power Left, Right Hook, Left Hook	Southpaw	ES	Repeat cycle 8 times
(8-move combo) Right Uppercut, Power Left, Right Hook, Power Left, Lateral Slip to Left, Right Jab, Right Jab, Power Left	Southpaw	ES	Repeat cycle 8 times

(16-move combo—just combine the last two combos in one longer combo)	Southpaw	ES	Repeat cycle 16 times
Right Jab, Right Jab, Power Left, Power Left, Power Right, Power Left, Right Hook, Left Hook, Right Uppercut, Power Left, Right Hook, Power Left, Lateral Slip to Left, Right Jab, Right Jab, Power Left			

Stimulation Stretch for Lower Body			
EXERCISE/STRETCH	**LENGTH OF TIME/ REPETITIONS**		
Squat Stretch	Perform the stretch once		
Ankle Circles	Perform the move once with each leg for 10 seconds		
Standing Calf Raise	Perform the exercise 25 times		
Jog (or jump) in place	Do for 30 seconds		
Tri Jumping Jacks	Perform the 3-part move once or twice for a total of 30–60 seconds		

ROUND ONE

AEROJUMP			
EXERCISE	**LENGTH OF TIME/ REPETITIONS**		
Boxer Skip	60 seconds		
Consecutive Double Under (Strive to do 10 in a row and do as many groupings of 10 as possible within the allotted time.)	180 seconds		

AEROSCULPT			
EXERCISE	**LENGTH OF TIME/ REPETITIONS**		
Aerofly (Level Four— Single-Leg Exchange) standing on left leg	30 reps		
Aerofly (Level Four— Single-Leg Exchange) standing on right leg	30 reps		

AEROBOX			
TYPE OF PUNCH	**POSITION**	**SPEED**	**DURATION**
(8-move combo) Left Jab, Left Jab, Power Right, Right Jab, Power Left, Power Right, Left Hook, Right Hook	Orthodox	ES	Do 2 cycles back-to-back (for a total of 16 punches). Rest for 4 seconds. Repeat the entire 16-punch/ 4-second rest cycle 8 times
(same as above)	Orthodox	FS	Repeat cycle 16 times—no rest in between
AEROJUMP			
EXERCISE	**LENGTH OF TIME/ REPETITIONS**		
Boxer Skip	60 seconds		
Consecutive Double Under (Strive to do 20 in a row and do as many groupings of 20 as possible within the allotted time)	180 seconds		

ROUND TWO

AEROBOX			
TYPE OF PUNCH	**POSITION**	**SPEED**	**DURATION**
(8-move combo) Left Uppercut, Power Right, Left Hook, Power Right, Lateral Slip to Right, Left Jab, Left Jab, Power Right	Orthodox	FS	Do 2 cycles back-to-back (for a total of 16 punches). Rest for 4 seconds. Repeat the entire 16-punch/ 4-second rest cycle 8 times
(same as above)	Orthodox	FS	Repeat cycle 16 times—no rest in between
AEROSCULPT			
EXERCISE	**LENGTH OF TIME/ REPETITIONS**		
Ankle Touch into Warrior	Do the exercise 8 times		

ROUND THREE

AEROBOX			
TYPE OF PUNCH	**POSITION**	**SPEED**	**DURATION**
(16-move combo—you're actually doing the same 8-move combos from Rounds One and Two back-to-back) Left Jab, Left Jab, Power Right, Right Jab, Power Left, Power Right, Left Hook, Right Hook, Left Uppercut, Power Right, Left Hook, Power Right, Lateral Slip to Right, Left Jab, Left Jab, Power Right	Orthodox	ES	Repeat cycle 4 times
(same as above)	Orthodox	FS	Repeat cycle 16 times—no rest in between

AEROJUMP			
EXERCISE	**LENGTH OF TIME/ REPETITIONS**		
Boxer Skip	60 seconds		
Consecutive Double Under (strive to do 20 in a row and do as many groupings of 20 as possible within the allotted time)	180 seconds		

ROUND FOUR

AEROBOX			
TYPE OF PUNCH	**POSITION**	**SPEED**	**DURATION**
(8-move combo) Right Jab, Right Jab, Power Left, Left Jab, Power Right, Power Left, Right Hook, Left Hook	Southpaw	ES	Do 2 cycles back-to-back (for a total of 16 punches). Rest for 4 seconds. Repeat the entire 16-punch/ 4-second rest cycle 8 times
(same as above)	Southpaw	FS	Repeat cycle 16 times

AEROSCULPT			
EXERCISE	LENGTH OF TIME/ REPETITIONS		
Aerofly (Level Four— Single-Leg Exchange) standing on left leg	30 reps		
Aerofly (Level Four— Single-Leg Exchange) standing on right leg	30 reps		

ROUND FIVE

AEROBOX			
TYPE OF PUNCH	POSITION	SPEED	DURATION
(8-move combo) Right Uppercut, Power Left, Right Hook, Power Left, Lateral Slip to Left, Right Jab, Right Jab, Power Left	Southpaw	FS	Do 2 cycles back-to-back (for a total of 16 punches). Rest for 4 seconds. Repeat the entire 16-punch/ 4-second rest cycle 8 times
(same as above)	Southpaw	FS	Repeat cycle 16 times—no rest in between

AEROJUMP			
EXERCISE	LENGTH OF TIME/ REPETITIONS		
Boxer Skip	60 seconds		
Side-Under (Fast)	Do 25 jumps (rest for 15 seconds); repeat 3 more times for a total of 100 jumps		

ROUND SIX

AEROBOX			
TYPE OF PUNCH	POSITION	SPEED	DURATION
(16-move combo— you're actually doing the same 8-move combos from Rounds Four and Five back-to-back) Right Jab, Right Jab, Power Left, Left Jab, Power Right, Power Left, Right Hook, Left Hook, Right Uppercut, Power Left, Right Hook, Power Left, Lateral Slip to Left, Right Jab, Right Jab, Power Left	Southpaw	ES	Repeat cycle 4 times

(same as above)	Southpaw	FS	Repeat cycle 16 times—no rest in between

AEROSCULPT			
EXERCISE	**LENGTH OF TIME/ REPETITIONS**		
Ankle Touch into Warrior	Do the exercise 8 times		

THE SLEEKIFY 5-MINUTE COOLDOWN			
Before you start, catch your breath by walking in place or side to side for 1 minute, or until your heart rate comes down.			
STRETCH	**LENGTH OF TIME/ REPETITIONS**		
Standing Tilt	Repeat twice to each side (hold each portion for 10 seconds)		
Back Bend/Forward Bend	Repeat 4 times back and forth (hold each portion for 10 seconds)		
Biceps-Forearm Stretch	Perform once with each arm (hold each stretch for 10 seconds)		
Shoulder-Triceps Stretch	Perform once with each arm (hold each stretch for 10 seconds)		
Sprinter's Calf Stretch	Perform the stretch 4 times with each leg for 10 seconds each time		
Kneeling Quad Stretch	Perform the stretch twice with each leg for 10 seconds		
Knee Hug	Perform the stretch once for 10 seconds		
Lying Hip-Glute Stretch	Perform the stretch twice with each leg for 10 seconds		
Hip Flexor Stretch	Perform the stretch once with each leg for 10 seconds		

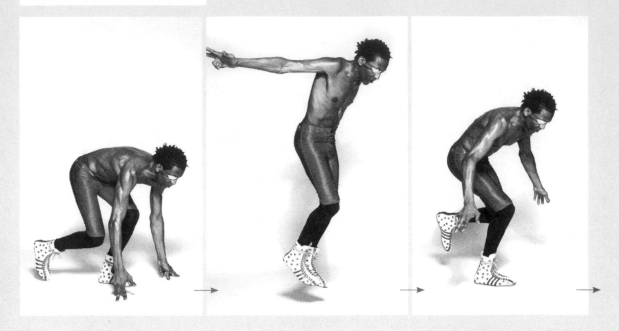

NEW AEROSCULPT MOVES

AEROFLY (LEVEL FOUR—SINGLE-LEG EXCHANGE)

START POSITION: Same as Aerofly (Level One)

THE MOVE: Keeping your left leg bent behind you, forcefully press yourself upward so that you pop off the floor. In midair, quickly sweep your arms out to the sides—like a pair of wings—then sweep them back in front of you so that your fingertips return to the start position.

The move is exactly like Aerofly (Level Three), only this time, instead of landing on the same foot you pushed off from (in this case, your right), you're going to switch legs

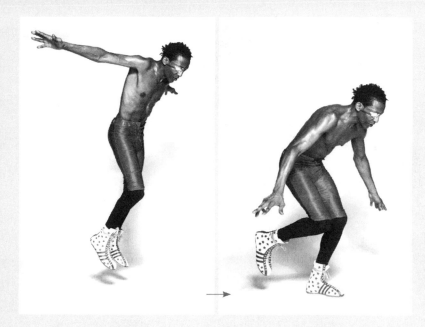

in midair so that you land on the opposite foot (in this case, your left). As you land, you should come down on the ball of your foot, then roll down to your heel.

The moment you land—right leg bent behind you, left foot on the floor, fingertips touching the floor—immediately squat down and repeat. Perform the exercise for as many repetitions as required, switching positions from balancing on your left foot to your right foot throughout the routine.

Aero-Tip

- Keep your quadriceps, glutes, calves, and core muscles flexed the entire time.

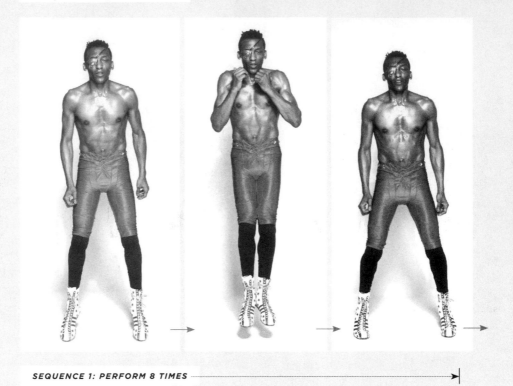

SEQUENCE 1: PERFORM 8 TIMES

ANKLE TOUCH INTO WARRIOR

START POSITION: Stand straight with your legs together, feet shoulder width apart, arms down by the sides of your thighs.

THE MOVE:

1. Without bending your knees, quickly jump straight up and bring your fists up by the sides of your face. In midair, touch your ankles and knees together at the top of the jump, then sweep them back out to the sides so that you land with your feet shoulder width apart. As you descend, bring your fists back down to the sides of your thighs. The movement should be fast—as if you're jumping rope—keeping your hands up by your face the entire time. Repeat the exercise eight times, then . . .

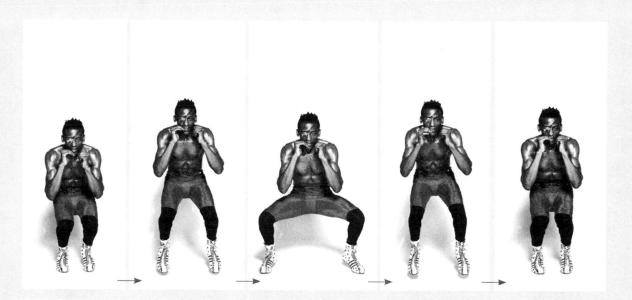

SEQUENCE 2: PERFORM 1 TIME

2.   Keeping your fists up by your face, space your feet close to each other and squat down until your butt is in line with your knees. Keeping your legs bent, quickly hop up so that your feet barely come off the floor and slide your feet apart from each other—your feet should feel as if they're skimming along the floor—so they end up wider than shoulder width apart. Immediately hop up again so that your feet barely come off the floor, but this time slide your feet in toward each other so that your knees touch. That's one repetition.

Aero-Tip

- Keep your quadriceps, glutes, calves, and core muscles flexed the entire time.

Past Aero-Moves to Expect

AEROBOX

- Jab
- Power Punch
- Uppercut
- Hook
- Lateral Slip

AEROJUMP

- Boxer Skip
- Double Under

AEROSCULPT

- Slow Aero Jack
- Slow Aero Shuffle
- Ankle Touch into Warrior

New Aero-Moves You Need to Know

AEROBOX

- Ali Lean
- Duran Drop
- Ali Shuffle
- O-Slip

AEROJUMP

- Aero Run (Knees Up)

- Slow Aero Downhill Squat
- Isometric Hold Squat

DAYS 25, 26, AND 27

NEW WEEK FOUR WARM-UP			
AEROBOX			
TYPE OF PUNCH	**POSITION**	**SPEED**	**DURATION**
(8-move combo) Left Jab, Left Jab, Power Right, Power Right, Power Left, Power Right, Left Hook, Right Hook	Orthodox	ES	Repeat cycle 8 times
(8-move combo) Left Uppercut, Power Right, Left Hook, Power Right, Lateral Slip to Right, Left Jab, Left Jab, Power Right	Orthodox	ES	Repeat cycle 8 times
(16-move combo—just combine the last 2 combos in 1 longer combo) Left Jab, Left Jab, Power Right, Power Right, Power Left, Power Right, Left Hook, Right Hook, Left Uppercut, Power Right, Left Hook, Power Right, Lateral Slip to Right, Left Jab, Left Jab, Power Right	Orthodox	ES	Repeat cycle 16 times
Stimulation Stretch for Upper Body			
EXERCISE/STRETCH	**LENGTH OF TIME/REPETITIONS**		
Standing Tilt	Repeat 4 times to each side (hold each portion for 10 seconds)		

Back Bend/Forward Bend	Repeat 4 times to each side (hold each portion for 10 seconds)		
Biceps-Forearm Stretch	Perform once with each arm (hold each stretch for 8 seconds)		
Shoulder-Triceps Stretch	Perform once with each arm (hold each stretch for 4–5 seconds)		

AEROBOX

TYPE OF PUNCH	POSITION	SPEED	DURATION
(8-move combo) Right Jab, Right Jab, Power Left, Power Left, Power Right, Power Left, Right Hook, Left Hook	Southpaw	ES	Repeat cycle 8 times
(8-move combo) Right Uppercut, Power Left, Right Hook, Power Left, Lateral Slip to Left, Right Jab, Right Jab, Power Left	Southpaw	ES	Repeat cycle 8 times
(16-move combo—just combine the last two combos in one longer combo) Right Jab, Right Jab, Power Left, Power Left, Power Right, Power Left, Right Hook, Left Hook, Right Uppercut, Power Left, Right Hook, Power Left, Lateral Slip to Left, Right Jab, Right Jab, Power Left	Southpaw	ES	Repeat cycle 16 times

Stimulation Stretch for Lower Body

EXERCISE/STRETCH	LENGTH OF TIME/ REPETITIONS		
Squat Stretch	Perform the stretch once		
Ankle Circles	Perform the move once with each leg for 10 seconds		
Standing Calf Raise	Perform the exercise 25 times		
Jog (or Jump) in Place	Do for 30 seconds		
Tri Jumping Jacks	Perform the 3-part move once or twice for a total of 30–60 seconds		

AEROBOX			
DRILL	**POSITION**	**SPEED**	**DURATION**
Ali Lean	Orthodox	FS	Repeat 64 times
Ali Lean	Southpaw	FS	Repeat 64 times
Lateral Slip	Orthodox	FS	Repeat 64 times
Lateral Slip	Southpaw	FS	Repeat 64 times
Duran Drop	Orthodox	FS	Repeat 64 times
Duran Drop	Southpaw	FS	Repeat 64 times
Ali Shuffle	Orthodox or Southpaw	FS	Repeat 32 times
O-Slip (Right)	Pyramid	ES	Repeat 8 times
O-Slip (Right)	Pyramid	FS	Repeat 32 times
O-Slip (Left)	Pyramid	ES	Repeat 8 times
O-Slip (Left)	Pyramid	FS	Repeat 32 times

ROUND ONE

AEROBOX			
TYPE OF PUNCH	**POSITION**	**SPEED**	**DURATION**
(5-move combo) Left Jab, Left Jab, Power Right, Power Left, Power Right	Orthodox	ES	Repeat cycle 8 times
(same as above)	Orthodox	FS	Repeat cycle 32 times—no rest in between
AEROSCULPT			
EXERCISE	**LENGTH OF TIME/ REPETITIONS**		
Slow Aero Downhill Squat	32 reps		
AEROJUMP			
EXERCISE	**LENGTH OF TIME/ REPETITIONS**		
Boxer Skip	180 seconds		
Double Under	Do 50 consecutive jumps		

ROUND TWO

AEROBOX			
TYPE OF PUNCH	**POSITION**	**SPEED**	**DURATION**
(3-move combo) O-Slip (Left), Left Hook, Power Right	Orthodox	ES	Repeat cycle 8 times
(same as above)	Orthodox	FS	Repeat cycle 32 times
(8-move combo) Left Jab, Left Jab, Power Right, Power Left, Power Right, O-Slip (Left), Left Hook, Power Right	Orthodox	ES	Repeat cycle 8 times
(same as above)	Orthodox	FS	Repeat cycle 32 times—no rest in between

AEROSCULPT			
EXERCISE	**LENGTH OF TIME/ REPETITIONS**		
Slow Aero Jack	32 reps		

AEROJUMP			
EXERCISE	**LENGTH OF TIME/ REPETITIONS**		
Boxer Skip	180 seconds		
Double Under	Do 75 consecutive jumps		

ROUND THREE

AEROBOX			
TYPE OF PUNCH	**POSITION**	**SPEED**	**DURATION**
(5-move combo) O-Slip (Right), Power Right, Left Uppercut, Power Right, Left Hook	Orthodox	ES	Repeat cycle 8 times
(same as above)	Orthodox	FS	Repeat cycle 32 times
(13-move combo) Left Jab, Left Jab, Power Right, Power Left, Power Right, O-Slip (Left), Left Hook, Power Right, O-Slip (Right), Power Right, Left Uppercut, Power Right, Left Hook	Orthodox	ES	Repeat cycle 8 times

(same as above)	Orthodox	FS	Repeat cycle 32 times—no rest in between

AEROSCULPT			
EXERCISE	**LENGTH OF TIME/ REPETITIONS**		
Slow Aero Shuffle	32 reps		

AEROJUMP			
EXERCISE	**LENGTH OF TIME/ REPETITIONS**		
Boxer Skip	180 seconds		
Double Under	Do 100 consecutive jumps		

ROUND FOUR

AEROBOX			
TYPE OF PUNCH	**POSITION**	**SPEED**	**DURATION**
(5-move combo) Left Jab, Duran Drop (Right), Right Uppercut, Left Hook, Power Right	Orthodox	ES	Repeat cycle 8 times
(same as above)	Orthodox	FS	Repeat cycle 32 times—no rest in between
(18-move combo) Left Jab, Left Jab, Power Right, Power Left, Power Right, O-Slip (Left), Left Hook, Power Right, O-Slip (Right), Power Right, Left Uppercut, Power Right, Left Hook, Left Jab, Duran Drop (Right), Right Uppercut, Left Hook, Power Right	Orthodox	ES	Repeat cycle 8 times
(same as above)	Orthodox	FS	Repeat cycle 32 times—no rest in between

AEROSCULPT			
EXERCISE	**LENGTH OF TIME/ REPETITIONS**		
Ankle Touch into Warrior	32 reps		

AEROJUMP			
EXERCISE	LENGTH OF TIME/ REPETITIONS		
Boxer Skip	180 seconds		
Double Under	Do 100 consecutive jumps		

ROUND FIVE

AEROBOX			
TYPE OF PUNCH	POSITION	SPEED	DURATION
(7-move combo) Ali Lean (Left), Ali Shuffle, Lateral Slip to Left, Left Uppercut, Left Hook, Power Right, Left Hook	Orthodox	ES	Repeat cycle 8 times
(same as above)	Orthodox	FS	Repeat cycle 32 times
(25-move combo) Left Jab, Left Jab, Power Right, Power Left, Power Right, O-Slip (Left), Left Hook, Power Right, O-Slip (Right), Power Right, Left Uppercut, Power Right, Left Hook, Left Jab, Duran Drop (Right), Right Uppercut, Left Hook, Power Right, Ali Lean (Left), Ali Shuffle, Lateral Slip to Left, Left Uppercut, Left Hook, Power Right, Left Hook	Orthodox	ES	Repeat cycle 4 times
(same as above)	Orthodox	FS	Repeat cycle 16 times— rest for 8 seconds in between each cycle
(same as above)	Orthodox	FS	Repeat cycle 16 times—no rest in between
AEROSCULPT			
EXERCISE	LENGTH OF TIME/ REPETITIONS		
Isometric Hold Squat	60 seconds		

AEROJUMP			
EXERCISE	**LENGTH OF TIME/ REPETITIONS**		
Aero Run (Knees Up)	180 seconds		
Double Under	Do 100 consecutive jumps		

THE SLEEKIFY 5-MINUTE COOLDOWN			
Before you start, catch your breath by walking in place or side to side for 1 minute, or until your heart rate comes down.			
STRETCH	**LENGTH OF TIME/ REPETITIONS**		
Standing Tilt	Repeat twice to each side (hold each portion for 10 seconds)		
Back Bend/Forward Bend	Repeat 4 times back and forth (hold each portion for 10 seconds)		
Biceps-Forearm Stretch	Perform once with each arm (hold each stretch for 10 seconds)		
Shoulder-Triceps Stretch	Perform once with each arm (hold each stretch for 10 seconds)		
Sprinter's Calf Stretch	Perform the stretch 4 times with each leg for 10 seconds each time		
Kneeling Quad Stretch	Perform the stretch twice with each leg for 10 seconds		
Knee Hug	Perform the stretch once for 10 seconds		
Lying Hip-Glute Stretch	Perform the stretch twice with each leg for 10 seconds		
Hip Flexor Stretch	Perform the stretch once with each leg for 10 seconds		

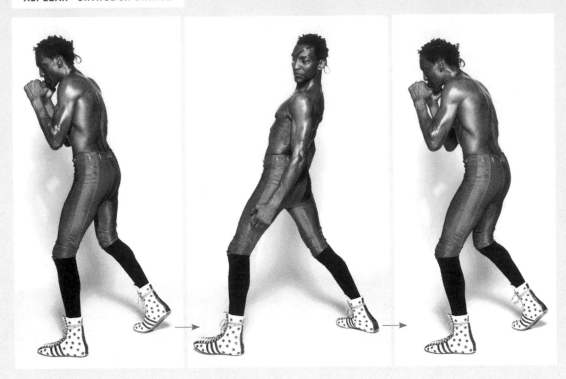

NEW AEROBOX MOVES

ALI LEAN

START POSITION: To lean to the left, start in Orthodox position—left foot forward, right foot back—with your fists up by the sides of your face. You should be on the ball of your right foot with your left foot flat on the floor, feet shoulder width apart.

THE MOVE: Keeping your eyes staring straight ahead (at your imaginary opponent), turn your head to the left slightly as you simultaneously lean back by taking a step backward with your right foot—your left foot will stay in place. As you lean, simultaneously drop your fists down to your sides. Step back into the start position—bringing your fists back up by the sides of your face—and repeat.

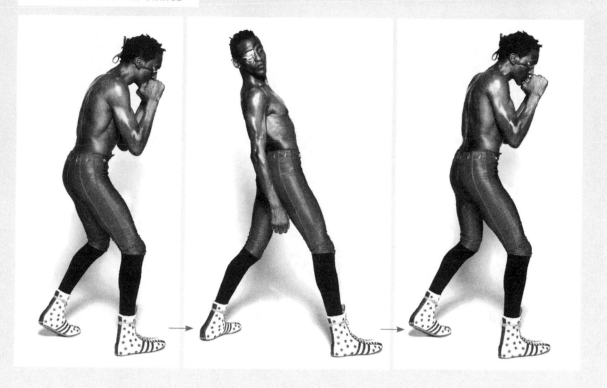

Aero-Tips

- When doing the Ali Lean to your right side, stay in an Orthodox stance and just turn your head to the right as you step back with your right foot.
- Don't look away from your opponent—keeping your eyes focused forward will prevent you from turning your head too far.

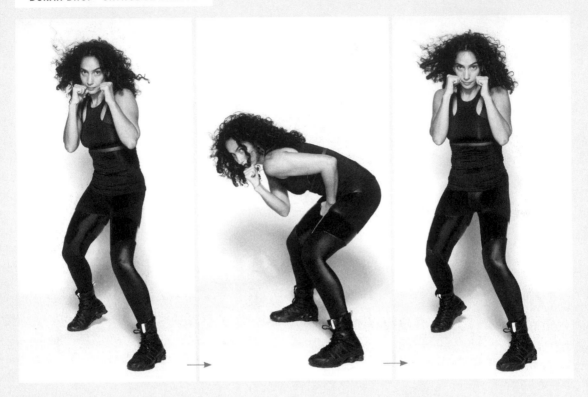

DURAN DROP

START POSITION: Start in Orthodox position—left foot forward, right foot back—with your fists up along the sides of your face, palms facing in. You should be on the ball of your right foot with your left foot flat on the floor, feet shoulder width apart.

THE MOVE: Bend your knees slightly as you twist your right shoulder farther behind you and drop to your right side. Simultaneously drop your left fist down and away from your face, keeping your right fist up by your face. (This maneuver is used to avoid an oncoming punch straight at you, so angle yourself so that a punch would go directly over your left shoulder.) Reverse the motion so you end up in the start position and repeat.

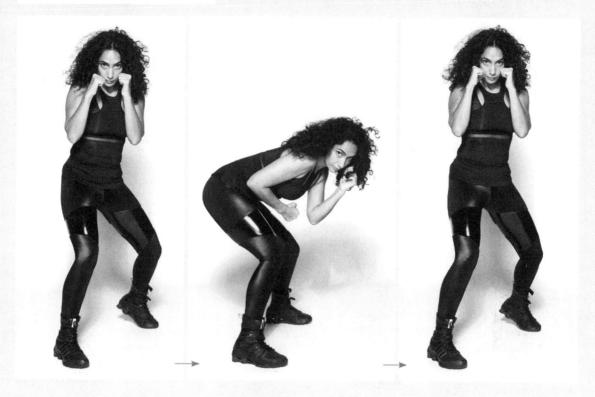

Aero-Tips

- When doing the Duran Drop to your left side, just switch into a Southpaw stance so that you can twist your left shoulder and drop to your left side.
- Don't look away from your opponent—keeping your eyes focused forward will prevent you from turning your head too far.

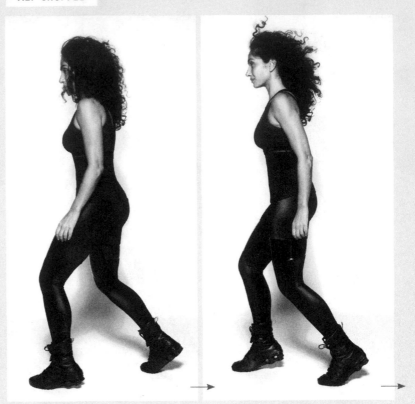

ALI SHUFFLE

ALI SHUFFLE

START POSITION: You can start in either an Orthodox position—left foot forward, right foot back—or Southpaw—right foot forward, left foot back. Either way, let your arms hang down by your sides, fists by your thighs.

THE MOVE: Keeping your arms down and your eyes facing forward (not at your feet), quickly shift your forward foot back while simultaneously sliding your back foot forward. Keep moving your feet as quickly as you can—left foot forward and right foot back, then right foot forward and left foot back—the entire time.

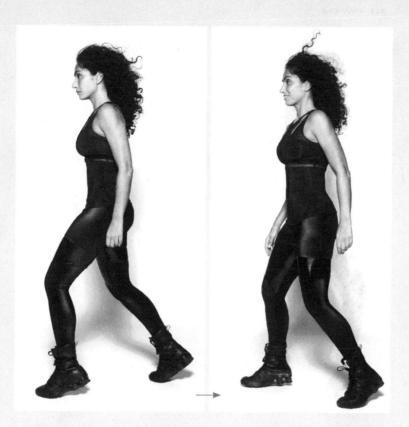

Aero-Tip

• Although you'll start with your back foot angled at either ten or two o'clock (depending on what stance you started from), the toes on both feet will stay pointing forward for the entire length of the drill.

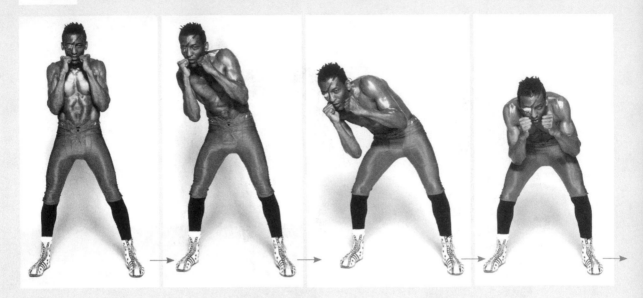

O-SLIP

START POSITION: Start in Pyramid position with your feet slightly wider than shoulder width apart, toes pointing forward, knees slightly bent (but muscles flexed). Your fists should be up along the sides of your face, palms facing in.

THE MOVE: To do this move, imagine you have pencils sticking out of your fists and you're about to draw two small circles in front of you.

To the left: Keeping your fists by your face and eyes facing forward, bend your knees so that your body drops down a few inches and then comes back up. As you go, simultaneously rotate your upper body to the left, then down, then under to the right in a circular motion.

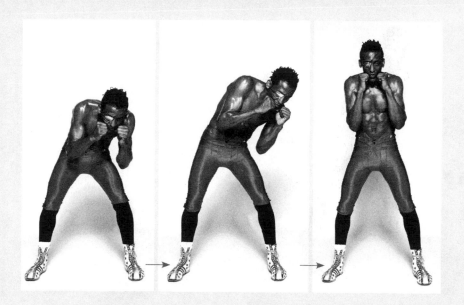

To the right: Maintaining the same posture, bend your knees so that your body drops down a few inches and then comes back up. As you go, simultaneously rotate your upper body to the right, then down, then under to the left in a circular motion.

Aero-Tip

- The drill should feel as if you're moving away from—and then underneath—an oncoming punch. If you're moving to the right, the bottom part of your right rib will move closer to your hip—then as you come up, your left rib releases from your left hip.

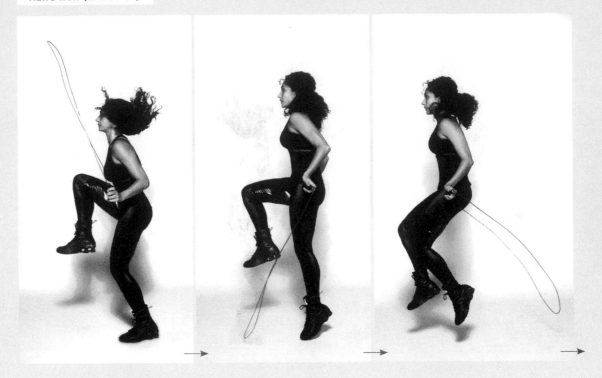

AERO RUN (KNEES UP)

NEW AEROJUMP MOVES

AERO RUN (KNEES UP)

This variation of the Aero Run is exactly the same, only instead of bringing one foot back as you jump over the rope with your opposite foot, you'll bring each knee up in front of you as high as you comfortably can.

START POSITION: Start by holding the rope at both ends—your arms should be down at your sides, palms facing forward. Step forward so that the middle of the rope is right behind your heels. Raise your right knee slightly up in front of you so that your right foot is off the floor.

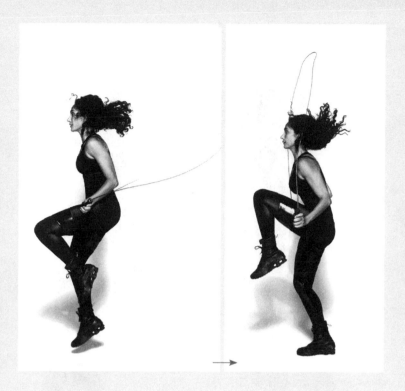

THE MOVE:

1.   Keeping your hands close to your body, begin turning the rope forward, rotating only from your wrists. Once the rope comes down toward your feet, take a tiny hop with your left foot to allow the rope to pass underneath you, as you raise your right knee up in front of you as high as you comfortably can.

2.   After the rope passes and your feet are in midair, switch feet by raising your left knee up in front of you, bringing your right knee back down so that you land on the ball of your right foot only. Once the rope comes down toward your feet again, take a tiny hop with your right foot to allow the rope to pass underneath you, as you raise your left knee up in front of you as high as you comfortably can.

3.   Continue alternating between jumping with your left foot only (right knee raised in front of you) and your right foot only (left knee raised in front of you) for the remainder of the exercise.

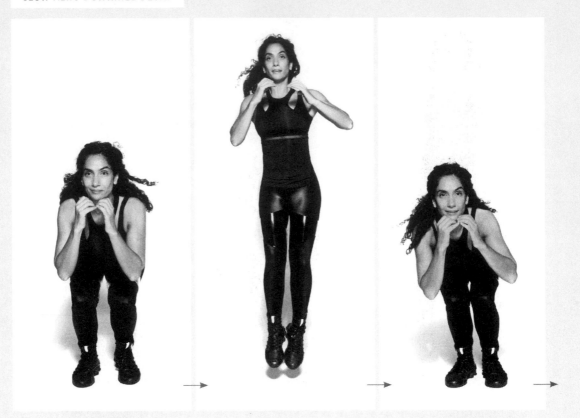

NEW AEROSCULPT MOVES

SLOW AERO DOWNHILL SQUAT

START POSITION: Stand straight with your legs together, knees and ankles touching—your fists should go up by the sides of your face just as if you were performing a basic squat.

THE MOVE: Keeping your legs together, squat down until your butt is in line with your knees, then slowly spring up off the floor—about half of the pace you used for the Downhill Squat on Days Four, Five, and Six—and laterally hop to your left. Land on the balls of your feet, then immediately repeat the exercise, this time hopping to your right. Continue to alternate from left to right throughout the exercise.

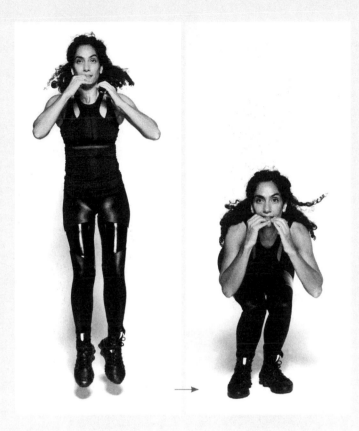

Aero-Tips

- Try to keep your heels off the floor throughout the entire move. Also, know that the higher you go, the slower your pace will be, so feel free to jump up as high as is comfortable. That may help your body move at a consistently slow tempo.
- Keep your quadriceps, glutes, calves, and core muscles flexed the entire time.

ISOMETRIC HOLD SQUAT

START POSITION: Stand straight with your feet shoulder width apart, arms extended out in front of you, palms facing the floor.

THE MOVE: Rise up on the balls of your feet, then squat down until your butt is in line with your knees. Pause at the bottom and hold yourself in this position—keeping your heels off the floor the entire time—for sixty seconds.

Aero-Tip

- Keep your quadriceps, glutes, calves, and core muscles flexed the entire time.

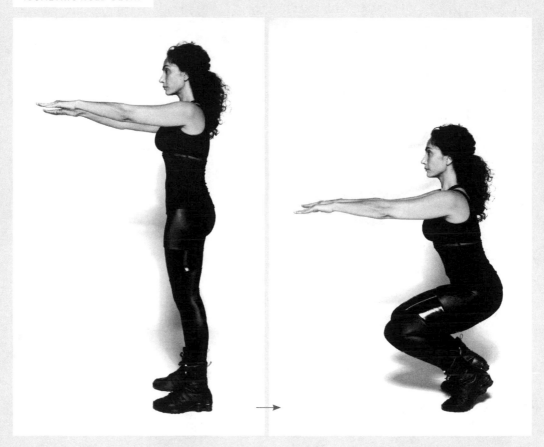

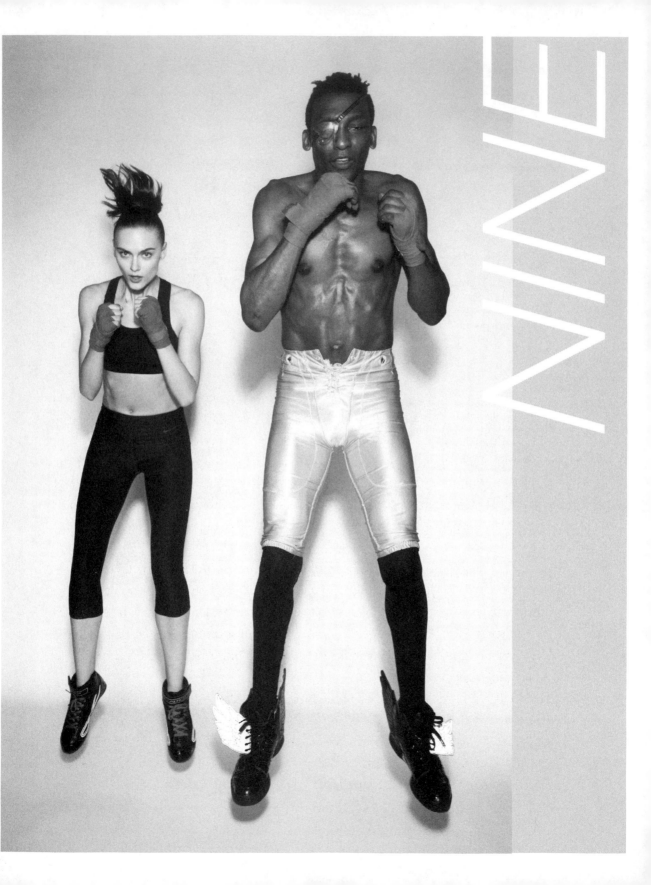

SLEEKIFY IN THE FUTURE

AFTER YOU REACH YOUR FITNESS GOALS THROUGH SLEEKIFY—AFTER YOU finally win your title—you have to defend it. And when it comes to staying lean, the fight is forever.

Defending the body you now have after completing the program can be a more difficult journey than the one you took to earn it. Sometimes that sense of accomplishment can cause you to let your guard down and do less, or quit and use something else that's less effective, simply because you feel you need to constantly mix things up for your body.

The good news is that Sleekify truly is the only program you'll ever need, because your muscles and mind will never completely master it. You can follow the Sleekify plan at any time to get yourself back on track, or continue to use it in perpetuity to help maintain your newly Sleekified physique for as long as you want to. However, once you've reached your weight loss goals using the program, you may need to modify it slightly to make it a lifelong fitness plan.

NOTE: If you haven't reached all of the fitness goals after twenty-eight days, the only thing I want you to do is repeat the twenty-eight-day program until you do. By finishing the program, you've created an atmosphere that's already helped you achieve amazing results. By keeping yourself within that atmosphere, you will force your body to continuously adapt until you've achieved all the results that the program can deliver. Each time you use Sleekify as prescribed, you will continue to improve on a daily basis until you earn your title.

You can also find more opportunities to grow stronger, fitter, and sleeker at www .aerospacehpc.com. I'll remain your cornerman, adding new ideas and techniques as we continue to learn together.

Now that you have the body you've always wanted, here's how to keep it, using these subtle tweaks to the Sleekify program.

SLEEKIFY: YOUR BODY—THE EXERCISE EDGE

Option #1: Change Sleekify from a four-week program to an

eight-month exercise experience

Although I have many clients who need to get in shape as quickly as possible—and perhaps that's you as well—in an ideal world, I prefer to spend a longer period of time working with a client so we can focus on each and every move for a longer duration.

If you don't have to race to be ready in a month—and if you're serious about being in the best shape of your life for the rest of your life—my dream-case scenario would be to have you use each of the eight three-day workouts for one month each.

For example, you would restart Sleekify using the workout prescribed for Days One, Two, and Three, but instead of moving on to the next workout after three days, you would continue using it for four straight weeks—six days a week (if you decide to take off the seventh day) or for the entire seven days. After four weeks, you would move on to the workout prescribed for Days Four, Five, and Six, repeat the same monthlong process, and continue to do so for a straight eight months.

What this will do is help you spend eight times longer honing every skill and perfecting every punch so each one begins to feel like second nature. Although the benefit of Sleekify is all in the effort, as you begin to struggle less and less with every punch, jump rope technique, and bodyweight exercise, the quicker you'll improve your coordination, cardiovascular capabilities, balance, and ability to burn off even more body fat.

Option #2: Modify the very last workout

As I mentioned in Week Four, the final week of the Sleekify program is the culmination of all of your hard work from the previous three weeks. It's the most complex week of the four, combining nearly every advanced technique and movement into one complete package. That said, if you chose to do nothing but the final week of Sleekify every week for the rest of your life, you could easily do that.

After finishing Sleekify, you may wonder why the final workout—Days 25, 26, and 27—asks you to perform all of your Aerobox maneuvers from only the Orthodox position (instead of repeating punch combinations from a Pyramid or Southpaw position as well). The answer is simple: Nine out of ten people are right-handed, and odds are, you are, too.

Although for the purposes of my exercise regime, I've asked you to throw punches from three different stances, fighters typically train and stay with one stance—the stance that's most natural for them. For 90 percent of all boxers—and 90 percent of the readers of this book—that natural stance is going to be Orthodox. Keeping you in an Orthodox stance for that final workout lets you feel what it is truly like to be a boxer.

However, if you're up for the challenge, you can always reverse the workout by performing it from a Southpaw stance and changing the direction of every punch and every lean of the body. Wherever you see an "L" or "Left," just change it to an "R" or "Right"— and vice versa. Using this simple tactic can make all of the Aerobox portions of the final Sleekify workout feel completely different to your muscles and mind.

Option #3: Improvise and Sleekify yourself

Even though I have created a twenty-eight-day program composed of eight individual routines that are a blend of exercises and drills designed to work your body from head to toe, that doesn't mean you have to stick to it to the letter.

As you become more experienced with all of the punches, jump rope techniques, and exercises within Sleekify, you can begin to take segments from each routine and create a customized workout of your own by mixing and matching your favorite Aerobox, Aerojump, and Aerosculpt moves.

Or, if you feel like trying other forms of exercise—such as cycling, running, and weightlifting, among others—you can also add any of the Aerobox, Aerojump, and Aerosculpt moves either in between sets or intervals, or before or after your workouts.

SLEEKIFY: YOUR DIET—THE NUTRITIONAL EDGE

All of the dietary rules that I spelled out in the nutrition chapter remain the same when you're looking to Sleekify for life. I still prefer that you eat only all-natural foods in smaller portions throughout the day, as well as stay away from any foods with preservatives, excess calories, and anything that your body cannot use as fuel.

However, once you've reached your ideal bodyweight, you can begin to ease back into eating more calories than the prescribed 1,200 to 1,500 calories per day. Instead, as you follow the program for life, your best bet is to eat the right number of calories to maintain your current bodyweight.

Knowing how many calories that amounts to is simple—all it takes is a calculator and your honesty. You see, your body requires only a certain amount of calories to maintain your current bodyweight each day. If you stick with that amount, your bodyweight shouldn't stray too far from where you are. But if you eat beyond that number each day, you can progressively begin to put a few pounds back on.

The easiest formula used by many nutritionists and trainers worldwide is this:

- If you're an active female (which you are if following the Sleekify exercise program), take your current weight—the weight you wish to stay at—then multiply that number by 12.
- If you're an active male (which again, you will be by following the Sleekify exercise program), take your current weight—the weight you wish to stay at—then multiply that number by 15.

The number you're left with is the amount of calories you should be eating each day to stay at your current bodyweight.

For example, if you're a woman who weighs 135 pounds, then you would multiply 135 x 12 (1,620), so the total amount of calories you should eat each day is around 1,620 to maintain your current weight.

If you're a man weighing 165 pounds, then you would multiply 165 x 15, so the total amount of calories you should eat each day is around 2,475 to maintain your current weight.

As you adjust to eating within these numbers, weigh yourself once a week in the morning, preferably on an empty bladder, to see if your weight fluctuates. If you find you are beginning to put on weight (wait for an increase of at least five pounds), you can revert back to the original 1,200 calories (for women) and 1,500 calories (for men) guidelines.

SLEEKIFY: YOUR MIND—THE MENTAL EDGE

What I love about Sleekify is that when it comes to the mental edge portion of the program, it's a philosophy that never needs to change—whether you're starting the routine for a second time or dedicating yourself to it forever. That's because all of the confidence-building skills essential to succeed with the program can be applied to all areas of your life.

In twenty-eight days, you've not only Sleekified your physique, you've unknowingly Sleekified your mind. You now have a sense of guidance and support you can use to improve every facet of yourself. Let your Sleekified physique serve as a reminder that anything is possible. Remember this: We are all the same inside and out—arms, legs, heart, brain, and so forth. But the bottom line is that what separates us is the ability to sacrifice. It's the willingness to do the hard work—the smart work—that separates the success from the regret. Sometimes you have to fight for what you want. I wish you success!

ACKNOWLEDGMENTS

SLEEKIFY™ WOULD NOT BE POSSIBLE WITHOUT THE ENERGY AND LESSONS OF many: my beautiful mom and incredible siblings, David, Sandra, and Tokunbo; my wife, Maryann, and children, Alex and Kayin; my business partner and friend, Leila Fazel; and all those who have taken the class over the years. I thank you all.

Special thanks to Alice and David Hunt, and Kelly and Jay Sugarman, as well as Felicia and Jeff Saferstein; Takeshi Uchida; my co-author, Myatt Murphy; Marnie Cochran, Jennifer Tung, Libby McGuire, Richard Callison, Joe Perez, and Nina Shield at Ballantine Books; George Karabotsos, Steve Perrine, and Dave Zinczenko at Galvanized Brands; and Josh Taekman, Ben Watts, Adriana Lima, Doetzen Kroes, Hugh Jackman, Angelo Dundee, Muhammad Ali, Jodi Cranston, Chris Gay, Rob Fernandez, Scott Marshall, and John Lederer. Also, special thanks to Zuzana Gregorova of DNA Models for gracing the back cover and appearing throughout this book.

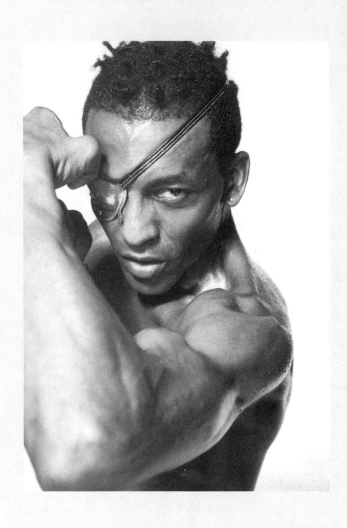

ABOUT THE AUTHORS

International fitness expert MICHAEL OLAJIDE, JR., is a former #1 ranked middleweight champion boxer and the co-founder, director of programs, and chief instructor at AEROSPACE High Performance Center in New York.

Dubbed the undisputed champion of boxing fitness, he also serves as private consultant to a host of celebrities (with past and present clients including Josh Hartnett, Mark Wahlberg, John Leguizamo, and supermodel Iman) and has acted as a consultant/choreographer for major movies and theatrical productions, including *Black Dahlia, Ali,* and *Subway Stories.* He has also been featured on major television networks and cable channels, including CBS, ABC, ESPN, FOX, and Nickelodeon.

aerospacenyc.com

MYATT MURPHY is the author of four popular exercise and nutrition books and is also an international journalist for more than forty-five magazines, including *Better Homes and Gardens, Cooking Light, Time,* and United Airline's *Hemispheres.*

myattmurphy.com

ABOUT THE TYPE

This book was set in Scala, a typeface designed by Martin Majoor in 1991. It was originally designed for a music company in the Netherlands and then was published by the international type house FSI FontShop. Its distinctive extended serifs add to the articulation of the letterforms to make it a very readable typeface.